CREDO

The Feldmár Institute makes use of the tools of philosophy, ethics and interpersonal phenomenology to approach human relationships. The Institute organises talks, workshops and groups to promote active engagement in intelligent and free communication that is unobstructed by shame.

www.feldmarintezet.hu

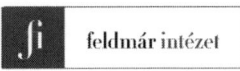 feldmár intézet

ANDREW FELDMÁR

CREDO

R.D. Laing and Radical Psychotherapy

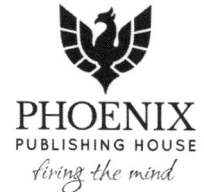

PHOENIX
PUBLISHING HOUSE
firing the mind

First published by HVG Könyvek, Budapest, in 2017 in Hungarian.

The English translation was published in 2021 by HVG Könyvek, Budapest, as a private limited edition to mark Andrew's 81st birthday.

Published in 2023 by
Phoenix Publishing House Ltd
62 Bucknell Road
Bicester
Oxfordshire OX26 2DS

The chapter entitled "A conversation with R.D. Laing" is reprinted with the permission of Robert Mullan

The chapter entitled "Shamanism, healing, and R.D. Laing" is reprinted with the permission of Francis Huxley

Translated by Julia Thornton

Edited by Soma Feldmár and Daniel Acs

Proofreading: Helen Douglas

British Library Cataloguing in Publication Data
A C.I.P. for this book is available from the British Library

ISBN-13: 978-1-80013-244-3

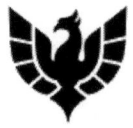

For Meredith

This means that play frees and distracts humanity from the sphere of the sacred, without simply abolishing it. The use to which the sacred is returned is a special one that does not coincide with utilitarian consumption ... This, however, does not mean neglect (no kind of attention can compare to that of a child at play) but a new dimension of use, which children and philosophers give to humanity.
Giorgio Agamben[1]

Hazard has conditioned us to live in hazard. All our pleasures are dependent on it. Even though I arrange for a pleasure, and look forward to it, my eventual enjoyment of it is still a matter of hazard. Whatever time passes, there is hazard. You may die before you turn the next page.
John Fowles[2]

Contents

Editor's Note

When the Feldmár Institute asked if I was interested in editing the English translation of my father's book, *Credo*, I immediately jumped at the opportunity. My father's work has been important to me for as long as I can remember, and I'm aware that he has helped many people get onto the path of "waking up," as he calls it. This has nothing to do with being "woke." It is simply about living one's life less asleep/as awake as possible. The member of the Feldmár Institute who started the project to get this book translated into English is Daniel Acs. He is the main or chief editor of this book. It is primarily his vision for this that guided everyone else, including me. However, for this English edition of *Credo*, we agreed it made the most sense for me to write the Editor's Note. In fact, way back at the beginning of this project, when all I had seen was the translation of the introduction, Daniel (Dani to friends, pronounced 'Donny') suggested that perhaps I could write some kind of opening piece for the book, sharing my personal connections to the events, stories, and histories told by my father. While agreeing to that, I also strongly encouraged him to write something for the Editor's Note, as well, because none of this would have happened without Daniel's initiative. In fact, because there's really the two of us here, it should be called the Editors' Note. I ended up asking him several questions to inspire him and get him writing.

Soma: Why do you think Andrew's work is important enough to share outside of Hungary?

Daniel: Andrew is one of the most popular and widely read psychotherapists in Hungary, and has been for the past 30 years. In 1956, at the age of 16, he immigrated to Canada all by himself. In 1992, he returned to Hungary as a recognised lecturer at the University of Debrecen. Since then, he has published 30 books in Hungarian. His first book, *The Rainbow of States of Consciousness*, is now in its third edition. The 2002 Hungarian documentary film about Andrew, *Is There Life before Death?*, was one of the very first films of Benedek Fliegauf, who later won, among other awards, a Silver Bear Grand Jury Prize, for his film *Just the Wind*, at the 2012 Berlin International Film Festival. Andrew is well-known in the field of psychedelic assisted psychotherapy to international audiences, having presented at numerous conferences on the subject. However, a deeper understanding of his views on psychotherapy, as well as the story of how he became the therapist he is, has only been available to Hungarian-speaking audiences up to this point.

Soma: And there are some organisations or groups, there in Hungary, that were formed because of Andrew's work, right?

Daniel: Yes, the Soteria Foundation was established in 1995, with guidance and regular hands-on supervision from Andrew, and became a pioneer of community psychiatric care in Hungary. They have operated daily clubhouses for those who live with psychiatric diagnoses, provided case management for people in the psychiatric system, and offered an employment service. Soteria was the first and only organisation in Hungary to operate an R.D. Laing-inspired shelter house. The house was active from 2012 to 2014. During that time, eight people lived there, with a maximum of five residents at a time. The Soteria Shelter Program is still in operation, without a physical house. Since 2015, the volunteers have been offering and providing company to people who need it, who need to spend time with someone and talk, without any expectations. I started volunteering for the program in 2012 and I was its leader for 7 years, starting in 2015.

In 2006, Andrew's colleagues and friends founded the Feldmár Institute, in Budapest, in order to popularise his theoretical and practical approach to psychotherapy. The Institute's mission is to work towards acquainting more and more people with the way of thinking and the "school" that Andrew represents in Hungary. Following the lineage of Aristotle, Winnicott, Wittgenstein, and Laing, the Institute promotes the spiritual wellbeing that can be experienced through free, honest, and unashamed communication. Through the Institute's programming, Andrew has been a regular guest, presenting lectures, running workshops, and teaching at Summer Universities throughout Hungary. The Story Circle in the Prison was a one-of-a-kind project by the Feldmár Institute in Balassagyarmat, a town north of Budapest, where Andrew worked directly with 65 prisoners. This project ran from 2011 to 2018 and achieved unique results in the field of reintegration.

I've been working at the Feldmár Institute as the spokesperson since 2017.

Soma: And why this book, *Credo*, and not one of the other many books of Andrew's in Hungarian?

Daniel: *Credo*, originally published in Hungarian in 2017, was launched at the Psychology–Philosophy Expo, an event put on by the Feldmár Institute, where the elite of Hungarian psychology and philosophy gave lectures and talked on stage, including Andrew. The two other great figures who were there, who are now sadly dead, are psychologist Tamás Vekerdy and philosopher Ágnes Heller. *Credo* was well received and became one of Andrew's most popular books. Tamás Vekerdy described *Credo* as an important insight not only into Andrew's life, but also into the world and era we currently live in.

Soma: You have a personal connection to this, too, don't you? It's not just other people in Hungary loving his work, it's very much you too, right?

Daniel: Absolutely. For me, the English translation of *Credo* is an important step towards allowing as many people as possible to meet Andrew's worldview, presented through the stories of his life and experiences. This worldview and his work have given me so much since 2012, when I first met him. Since then, Andrew has been a role model for me, an idol to be overthrown, a professional mentor, a podcast co-host, and, above all, a person with whom it is always good to talk. He is a master who is spontaneous, but most often tactful; who is honest, but always loving; and who is always worth paying attention to.

Soma: An idol to be overthrown? Can you explain that a bit, please?

Daniel: I mean, he quickly became the Perfect Man for me, someone I could worship but not actually know like another person. I was so afraid of him. I felt like I would die of shame if he judged me. It was difficult to know that if he really mistreated me, I could stand up for myself. I hated that I felt so nervous around him. I projected a lot of things onto him, and didn't know who he really was. But my frustration and desire to know him were bigger than my fear, so I grabbed every opportunity I could to spend time with him. Over the last ten years, the two of us have been involved in several projects together, including a 100-part podcast series, which was later published as a book. I have since become a therapist myself, and Andrew is my supervisor and colleague. The nervousness is gone, but the love and respect for him is not, neither is the joy that I can spend time with him and learn from him.

Daniel's wonderful explanation quickly recalled two experiences I've had regarding my father that kind of go together. One of them is just the fact that he's my father: it's not exactly "an experience". For my entire childhood, he was the one in control. He had the power, he made the rules, with my mother, of course, and he enforced the repercussions. As I grew up, he started to become more and more successful where we lived and in the social circles our family was part of. At times, it felt as though I was Andrew Feldmár's daughter more than I was Soma, just me. One of the things that has become a constant in my life, since then, is practising and remembering that his way is one way, and not necessarily the right way, or my way.

The other experience, which makes me smile and sometimes even laugh when I remember it, happened when I encountered people during my teen and young adult years who openly worshipped my father, with zero notion of changing or overcoming it. It was summertime, I was probably in my mid-teens, so it was maybe 1988, and I was heading to Cortes Island from Vancouver on my own. That meant taking a Greyhound-style bus from downtown Vancouver to the ferry over to Nanaimo, and getting another bus up Vancouver Island to Campbell River. Once there, I'd walk over to the ferry terminal, get my ticket, and hitch a ride across the next island with someone in a car going all the way to Cortes. It was 1984 when my father organised his first retreat at Hollyhock, and he writes about it in his introduction to this book. There were many more highly attended and successful retreats and workshops he gave there, over the years. Hollyhock was the only reason my family and I came to Cortes Island in the first place. This one summer, I got a ride with three women who were on their way to the Hollyhock retreat centre on Cortes. The three women and I started to get to know each other a bit, and when they found out who I was, one of them said, incredulously, "YOU'RE Andrew Feldmár's DAUGHTER?!" Another said, "Wow!" And the third woman said, and this is the zinger, "I want my children to grow up to be JUST LIKE YOU!" In an adolescent attempt to burst their "Andrew bubble", I recounted a number of moments when my father's frustration had got the better of him, and he yelled some pretty crazy things at me. One very strange thing he used to yell at me, which somehow never worked because he'd never do such a thing, and never made me stop crying, was, "Stop CRYING or I'll FLATTEN your FACE!" I thought that would get them, but no matter. The three women continued to watch me as though I were some rare shiny specimen of something.

The experience and work of editing the English translation of this book have been amazing in multiple ways. As someone who has been involved in writing, language, and books for many years (all my education has been in writing and literature: I am a published poet and have a PhD in English), it had been slightly disappointing to me that only one of Andrew's Hungarian books has some English in it: the bilingual edition of his poems. I couldn't read any of his other books, and they were the ones I wanted to read. I knew I wanted to be involved if any of his books were ever going to come out in English, but I never expected this to happen during his lifetime. Being able to work on one of his books, and this book in particular, while my father is still alive, so to actually work WITH him on the English edition of *Credo*, has been thrilling, intense, educational, and even somewhat transformative. The first two chapters of this book, the "Introduction" and "Ruptures", provide some of the more general conceptual and experiential histories that have shaped my father's being and beliefs. The time span covered goes from his childhood to much more recent history, meaning I was, during some of those moments, present and alive. I remember our very first trip to Cortes Island and Hollyhock, to check it all out and make sure my father wanted to hold his workshop there. I remember the big feelings, high energy, tension, and vivacious atmosphere around that first workshop my father organized. The community and other families around Hollyhock became an important part of my later childhood and teen years. Cortes Island was my adolescent coming-of-age dreamland, and now, over 30 years later, it has become my home. What a gift it has been to read Andrew's experience of that workshop and to learn how important it was for his life and career.

The longest chapter of this book comes from notes my father took during the year (August 1974–August 1975) he worked and studied with Ronnie and the Philadelphia Association. I was not quite a year and a half old, and my brother had just turned four, when my family relocated to London, England for a year, so my father could work and study with R.D. Laing. I don't have any conscious memories from that time, but I do have many memories of Laing, whom I always knew as Ronnie, and some of the other people Andrew met and became colleagues with during that important year in London. In fact, Francis Huxley became such a close friend of our family that he was like an uncle to me. Ronnie wasn't like that, though. He didn't engage with my brother and I the same way Francis did. The other two people from back then I've met are Paul Zeal and Leon Redler. The memories I have of Paul are from a very particular summer he came to visit, when we took a trip to a little place called Goat Island. I remember my father plucking sea urchins out of the ocean, from the canoe, and sucking out the alive edible parts. Paul, in my memory, was energetic, curious, and easy for me to be around as a kid. Leon ended up becoming a closer friend of my father's, so I have more memories of him from my childhood, as well as his family. One of his daughters is a similar age to me, and there were a couple times we played together during visits. Leon was fun to listen to and watch. He was often rather animated, red-faced with laughter, exciting, and occasionally a wee bit scary to me when I was young. The most vivid memories I have of Ronnie are listening to him play our white stand-up piano when he came to visit, usually drunk; watching him question and upset my older brother to tears at a restaurant, which I secretly relished; and once, when I was maybe 13 or 14, watching him try to make coffee in our kitchen one morning, when suddenly, his pants dropped to the floor. He was not wearing any underwear. We were both surprised, but neither of us made a noise; he simply pulled up his pants and continued. I often wish I had paid more attention back then, that I had known then, and even before, when I was younger, the importance and relevance of some of the adults I spent time with.

In some ways, I have learned more about my father since beginning this project in early 2020 than I have being his daughter for 50 years. The second chapter, "Ruptures", is the most autobiographical part of the book and tracks some of the more impactful and important events in my father's life, according to him. Reading through this section, editing it, and then going over it again with my father, taught me things about him and his past experiences, about my Hungarian grandparents, and about his history with my mother that I didn't know before. Working through the "Journal Entries" chapter also taught me a lot about my father. This time, it was in relation to his work with Ronnie and the therapy, training, and guidance he received during that year. It was like going through his university notebooks and his private diary at the same time. One of the most amazing discoveries for me is that there are things he learned back then that he has held onto to this day. I don't just mean concepts, ideas, and beliefs. There are those, of course. But what surprised me is there are phrases, turns of phrase, and sentences that have, over the past 48 years, remained, word for word, in my father's mind and work. I'd be reading along, doing my editing work, and suddenly a phrase would pop up from my childhood! Ha-ha! It was like some sort of bizarre psychological time travel! But it does go to show that when someone learns something that resonates as a truth in their being and life, it can remain for the rest of their lives. I'm still surprised that the words are the same, but my father used to write lots of poetry and he studied psycholinguistics, so perhaps I shouldn't be so surprised that he hung on to the words. Words have always been important for him. This editing work has shown me more personal truths and stories from and of my father than anything ever before. While Andrew has always been available to me as a father, friend, guide, staunch supporter, and defender, he has rarely, if ever, divulged himself to me. I think this is partly because of his naturally shy demeanour, partly because of his practice and beliefs as a father, and partly simply a result of his profession as a therapist. It is, and has been, more than I could have imagined, and I am aware that such opportunities for fathers and daughters to work together and share like this are few and far between. I cannot possibly express how grateful I am for this. Or, by saying that, I suppose I express it as much as I can.

The only things I'd like to say about the actual editing and some of the choices I made have to do with the use of personal pronouns and the notes at the end of the book. At one point, I counted all the notes I added to the manuscript, on top of the ones from the original Hungarian edition, and, though I forget the exact number, it was somewhere in the vicinity of 180. Part of the reason I did this is my intense and thorough academic training (cite! cite! cite!); part of it is because one of my beliefs about thinking, thought, and ideas is that thinking is only possible in conversation and company, so it's important to show that; and, finally, because I am committed to providing the readers of this book as many opportunities to follow Andrew's intellectual journeys as possible. That commitment comes from my own way of reading, and knowing that if I were reading this book, I would want all those references and all those sources. It was quite the journey for me doing all the research, asking Andrew hundreds of questions, writing so many notes, and learning so so much! Speaking of learning, one of the cool things I learned is that the Hungarian language doesn't use gendered pronouns; it's a gender-neutral language. I love that. When I started editing the translated manuscript, I discovered that the translator had gendered all anonymous adults with the pronoun "he" and all anonymous children and babies with the pronoun "she." I actually had to remind myself that it was the translator doing her best to follow traditional conventions, and not Andrew being oddly sexist in his writing. Since I know my father is not sexist in the least, and I, myself, have no single gender identity, I made the editing choice to use the gender-neutral singular pronoun we have in English, "they," for all otherwise anonymous individuals, regardless of age. While I know this is a relatively recent occurrence in English, there is a precedent for it, both in older versions of English and in other related languages.

Soma Feldmár, Cortes Island, Canada, March 2023

PREFACE. *By Alphonso Lingis*

"Every child wants to cure their parents, so they can be loved in a way that is good for them. But there are some children who don't succeed. Maybe they are the ones who become therapists," Andrew Feldmár says. He tells of being born of Jewish parents in Hungary during the Second World War; when he was three and a half years old, his parents were taken separately to labour camps and he was hidden in a Christian family. When the war ended, his parents were divorced, and, five years old, he was taken by his now possessive and cruel mother. When he was sixteen, he escaped Hungary and his mother to Canada. He studied mathematics in graduate school. After a divorce and a time of deep depression, Andrew underwent intensive psychoanalysis, until he realised he could be a better therapist than his analyst. He worked five years in a mental health clinic with troubled young children. Then, aged 34, he went to London to train under Ronnie Laing.

In 1951–53 Ronald David Laing, on his first military assignment after finishing medical school, worked in the Royal Victoria Hospital and the Catterick Military Hospital with shell-shocked soldiers. He was horrified by the cruelty of the insulin-shock and electroconvulsive treatments, the strait jackets and padded cells, and the issuing of powerful and ill-tested drugs he was enjoined to inflict. He was ordered to even exaggerate the cruel treatments to the patients, in order to detect malingerers.

He came to believe that a psychotic crisis is an experience in which the patient is dealing with a past trauma, perhaps a double-bind situation, and that this may issue in profound insights for the patient. The breakdown may be a breakthrough to transformative experience. There is the opportunity for the therapist also to learn important insights about living, about the world, about the cosmos from the patient. There is also the risk that there could be something going on in the patient that may infect or poison the therapist.

Andrew spent a year in London. He attended seminars at the Philadelphia Association, read books, underwent psychotherapy by Laing and, with Laing's supervision, began to practice therapy. He gives us to read the journal he kept. Laing opened Andrew to philosophy; Francis Huxley to anthropology: to myths, healers, shamans. Andrew's enthusiasms for all the ideas that glittered before him and also his admiration for the courage and kindness of the therapists are intense. He recounts, too, his doubts and anxieties, and the month, half through the year, when he sunk into bewilderment and depression. He tells of his fears in visiting the shelters where psychotics and schizophrenics are unsupervised.

He looks on a patient who breaks all the windows, eats off the floor and shits everywhere. The whole house is dirty, smells of shit, it invites one to not look after it, to vandalise it, All the others have moved out. Andrew reflects that this place is not healing of anything. But later he learns that this patient came to his senses, was cured and moved out. It took another year. "What a miracle!"

Andrew's admiration for Laing's vast intellect and for his patience, courtesy and generosity has not faded in the intervening fifty years. But, at the time, Andrew also recognised times when Laing was beset with alcoholism, depression and doubt.

Andrew includes a text by Francis Huxley explaining how Laing had the temperament of a shaman but his psychotherapy was not shamanism, and recounting the complexity of his personality and practice. Andrew also includes an interview where Laing explains himself.

Then Andrew, after fifty years of practice, writes of some of his thoughts about the disturbances people suffer and what effective therapy is. What he writes contains a response to an objection many people have, that psychotherapy conducts people into a long and tedious self-absorption. Unless one is paralysed by anxiety or depression, or suicidal, these people are repelled by the prospect of spending months, years, scrutinising dreams and memories of details of one's childhood. But Andrew peremptorily denies that psychotherapy has knowledge of oneself as its goal. At most, one would then envision oneself as the object family and social authorities envision. "'Work on yourself!' prevents revolutions, discourages solidarity and creates the false ideal that I should be able to rise above my circumstances, no matter how oppressive, injurious or crazy-making they are." It is coming to know others that is liberating.

Many people are afraid to acknowledge cruel and scandalous thoughts that come to them. A therapist demystifies fears and encourages courage. He or she encourages the patient to identify habits and fears that are preventing the patient from acting. Habits can be broken; when Andrew began therapy with Laing, he drew up a long list of all his habits, and found he was able to break the undesirable ones. "Therapy has ended when the patient becomes so busy that they forget about the session", when projects that are important to them: work, family, friendships, and the world "become more important than therapy."

Andrew Feldmár's book engages those of us who are psychotherapists or patients undergoing therapy and also those of us who are not. For we do accompany others who are going on their own path as we seek to go on a path of our own. We accompany many people who live their lives energetically and happily. But we also accompany others who are suffering. To help them is to help them find their own path. And we accompany others who are going nowhere, who are dying.

Alphonso Lingis

INTRODUCTION

In 1984, Ronald (Ronnie) D. Laing, Francis Huxley and Leon Redler from London, and David Bakan, together with his wife and colleague Mildred, from Toronto, came to Hollyhock, a retreat and learning centre on Cortes Island, in British Columbia, Canada. I organised a five-day workshop for forty people called "Pain, Suffering and the Possibility of Healing". This was the first time in my life I organised such a major workshop independently, and it proved to me that I could actually do it. I had discovered a new world, without biting the dust in the process. I got the people together, everyone came, everything worked and I managed to pay all the bills and even make some money. More than thirty years have passed since then, and I have organised many workshops – but this first one was the ship that broke the ice.

The workshop was greatly significant in my life for another reason, too. I invited a very diverse group to lead the workshop: on one hand, the two Bakans, who were deeply religious Jews; on the other hand, Huxley and Laing, who were Pagans. Redler and I were in the middle, although we were both Jewish by birth.[1] From goodness knows where, David Abram turned up unexpectedly – a vagabond and magician at the time, besides his day job as a philosopher.[2] He was very amusing, making coins disappear then conjuring them up again. He even pushed a coin through my hand. His jugglery made all parties laugh, which lightened the heavy atmosphere created by sparks of tension caused by the enmity between Jews and Pagans. It all started with Huxley telling us how he was burdened with dark sadness for a year after his father passed away. Then one day he looked up in the sky and saw seven ravens. Exactly seven. Three were flying in one direction and four flew across the other way. He knew and felt right away that his mourning was over. That was the sign, and he felt incredibly relieved. Mildred Bakan immediately retorted that it was just a psychotic defence, a superstition, and that one couldn't just put an end to the grief caused by the death of a parent. She said she would feel the absence of her mother as long as she lived. Huxley grew extremely angry and told Mildred indignantly that she would never become his psychotherapist, and she should have kept her opinions to herself. From then on, those two didn't talk to each other. Huxley was swearing – Jews don't like nature, he said – and David Bakan took me aside to warn me about the antisemitism of Laing and Huxley, warning that I didn't stand a chance against them. Why was I so friendly with them, could I not see how dangerous they were? Tensions mounted. Conflicting styles, beliefs, philosophies and ethics clashed, reverberating throughout the atmosphere. Bakan didn't trust either Huxley or Laing; he considered them devoid of ethics because the way they spoke and thought expressed the idea that God is, or the gods are, hiding in the trees, the birds, the air, in the entirety of nature. According to the Bakans' Jewish faith and ethics, there is only one God, their God. They believed that the Nazis also started off with "God exists in everything", and they were terrified of this nature worship. Is monotheism ethical and the idea that gods exist in everything unethical? I found all this completely open hostility really exciting and liberating. I didn't have to worry about or protect either side. I had learned from them, and I had a good practice of being honest and spontaneous even when it was unpleasant. Naturally, everyone sensed the tensions, and some people were scared because the situation reminded them of their parents arguing. My friendships with Huxley, Laing and the Bakans, however, remained intact. It seemed like my role was to bridge gaps and connect worlds that felt mutual dislike and hostility. I was able to be friends with both worlds, there on the island. Somehow, I possessed this talent. I am a mediator. I exist halfway between traditional Jewish ethics and Pagan, Celtic tradition, just like between my mother and my father. My parents had divorced; my father lived in Pest, and I lived in Buda with my mother. I can see myself as a young boy, plodding along Margit Bridge from one to the other, always there and back, across, then across again. I am the connection, like the corpus callosum between the two cerebral hemispheres.

I was born in Budapest in 1940, a child of a Jewish couple, right in the middle of Hitler's Nazism and antisemitic persecution. They argued about whether or not I should have a circumcision ritual. My mother thought I shouldn't be stigmatised, and maybe we could even hide the fact that I'm Jewish, and my father was worried that God might punish us if we were not good Jews. Actually, neither of them identified as a Jew; they considered themselves Hungarian, but by that time it didn't make any difference. By 1940, the right to determine one's own identity had been lost. My parents didn't speak Yiddish, they didn't really know any Hebrew words, they couldn't recite a prayer properly and they didn't go to synagogue. They were completely assimilated. It was a terrible surprise for them that suddenly they had to wear the yellow star. They didn't want to wear it and didn't wear it, but I was a little boy who really liked it, and I demanded that they sew it on my clothes.

Later on, something – I haven't got the faintest idea what – strongly attracted me to the Celts, the historical ancestors of the Irish and Scottish people. Maybe it was the inextinguishable patriotic spirit of fighting for freedom that's so similar to Hungarians, or the ethos of being oppressed that caught me; I don't know. Patricia Wilensky, my friend and colleague, is of Irish descent. Laing, my teacher and mentor, was Scottish. They and other Celtic thinkers and scientists have always had a greatly liberating influence on me, to this very day. Somehow, through their world, I got in touch with an ancient European Pagan tradition. Zalman Schachter-Shalomi[3] says that God is a pot of boiling water, and each escaping droplet is a new life, a human being. The drop appears, darts up, then falls again and becomes part of the whole once more in the pot until it appears again in another construction. Death, then, is taking a dip in God. In this cycle, God and His creations are one; God exists in everything. This is a perfectly Pagan cycle, even though a rabbi explained it. It seems like the divisions aren't so clear after all.

Huxley and Laing weren't particularly understanding and tactful during the Cortes Island workshop. Huxley swore, called Pakistani people "Pakis", made crude and outrageous jokes about such things, and sometimes even about Jews. But I know he never would have bullied me because of my Jewishness, just as he wouldn't bully anyone else. The Bakans were paranoid about how Laing's and Huxley's company put me in mortal danger. It was as if they didn't want to lose me; they didn't want to abandon me to marauding Pagans. In other words, the island saw the conflict brewing between Jews and Pagans. In my life, however, there are Christians between the two. A Christian woman named Irén Igaz saved my life. In Hungarian, *igaz* means "true" or "righteous". Risking her own life and the life of her family, she hid me for a year and a half, during the most rotten, depraved Arrow Cross frenzy.[4] This set up the path I would take to become a therapist. A stranger protected and looked after me, and now I am the protective stranger present in the lives of so many perplexed and wounded people.

So, that summer, on Cortes Island, is very significant. It was there and then that I realised, while I don't know how to deal with my Jewishness, I don't feel at home in the other world either. I was travelling, walking back and forth, just like I do now, between two languages and between my two home countries: Canada and Hungary.

After the workshop, Laing took me aside and congratulated me, in private, for conducting my own psychotherapy so publicly and for making money in the process. He knew that what had happened there, on the island, was a reflection of the split in my soul, and it was such a smart move to involve them in this psycho-drama. At that point, I realised that wasn't the only time this had happened. I did, and do, this constantly. I didn't actually have therapy for an extended period of time; first, I had five sessions a week for nine months, and second, I had 8–9 hours a week for a year with Laing in London. It wasn't a long time, but it was enough for me to, in Laing's words, be able to "market my pathology". Being a therapist is one of the methods. I heal myself publicly because the therapy I am doing for other people cures me as well. This book is also therapy for me. It is therapy because there is resistance in me to writing a book. I'd rather do anything else to avoid it: sharpen pencils, make coffee or go for a walk. It seems I am still struggling with things. I don't want to remember everything. I don't want to believe that I am worthy and interesting. I am scared of exposing myself in case I get hurt or people won't like me. But I go against the grain. I go against my father, as well, who taught me that, for survival, one must always crawl like a worm to wherever the powerful may be, and grovel, and that one should be invisible and unnoticeable. I expose myself in order to stop being a stranger.

My friend Alphonso Lingis, an Anglo-Saxon representative of European ethics, travels widely and has a lot of personal experience as a stranger, with strangers. Once, his legs became paralysed in India, and he couldn't move. Somehow, he crawled out of the tent he slept in and just waited for something to happen. A stranger happened to pass that way and, would you believe it, he dragged him to the seashore, took him across the bay to the other side with a catamaran that happened to be there, rushed him to the hospital with a taxi, and then disappeared. Lingis couldn't even say thank you. Lingis also told me about a young man who wanted to travel around Europe, but just as he set off on the train, he was robbed of all his possessions. In complete desperation, he phoned his parents from the station and told them, weeping, what had happened. His parents reassured him they would send him some money somewhere, just enough for him to return home. A man standing on the other side of the phone booth went up to him and explained that he couldn't help but overhear the conversation. He gave him five thousand dollars right there and then, with a "there you go, no need to thank me" and disappeared. You see, one stranger robbed him and another stranger helped him out. Another time, Lingis sat in a taxi at the airport of an Indian city, and the driver asked him straight away if he wanted some hash. "I can give you now," he said. Lingis thought for a moment. "Why not," he said, and "yes." The driver took him straight to the police station. "I've brought a drug addict foreigner," he said. The policeman gave him back the hash, and Lingis spent a few days in jail before the consulate managed to free him. Somehow, Lingis likes to be alone in the world, dependent on strangers. He is over eighty years old now, but to this day, he exposes himself to strangers, to the other, and this is sometimes good, sometimes bad. But he can't pick and choose his experiences, rather, he is grateful for *having* experiences at all. If one overprotects oneself, one never finds out that the other, the stranger, can actually be of help. We can only experience this by exposing ourselves. Making myself vulnerable, being helpless, and the other still not hurting me is a healing moment. It is not sufficient to contemplate this; one has to experience it.

My Jewishness makes the issue of being a stranger very significant; after all, my foundational experience in life is that "I am different". We thought we were Hungarians, but then it turned out we were different, Jewish, strangers. "Hey, you know us, don't you? It's us!" We could say this all we liked. Our voice was not heard, like in a bad dream. Emmanuel Levinas[5] gives a clear explanation of the stranger just being a terrible illusion: the moment the other has a face, I am indebted to him. No one born of a mother can possibly be a stranger. The stranger one has to be scared of is not a reality. Levinas realised this after the concentration camps. We have to wake up from this idea that there are us and them. We are unified by having a face. By looking into the other's face, I position them above myself. In Martin Buber's world[6], I and the other are equal, but Levinas declares the other to be more important than the self. I designate Levinas's philosophy "maternal ethics", even if it sounds silly, because in a mother's consciousness, the child is more important than herself. This is the foundation. This is the starting point, and this is where we return. How can one live with this ethics? If one is not in an emergency, one can definitely rely on Rabbi Hillel's triple rule: "If I am not for myself, who will be for me? And if I am only for myself, what am I? And if not now, when?"[7] Because I can only give to the other if I am alive: if I snuff myself out trying to help the other, then I can't help them. Mothers also know that they have to look after themselves because the child is in deep trouble if the mother dies. The worst thing that can happen to a patient is if their therapist burns out or dies on them, either by losing interest or actually dying.

When I arrived in London at the age of 34, I visited all the prominent guys working in the Philadelphia Association at the time.[8] I saw Ronald D. Laing, Francis Huxley, Leon Redler, Hugh Crawford and John Heaton. I discussed my desires, opportunities and hopes with them, as well as the fastest way for me to get the most from them. Even at that time, 1974–75, London was expensive. I was poor, so I had to find the shortest possible way to lay my hands on all the knowledge and experience that could benefit me. I told them of my desire to discover something new, to uncover something no one had ever thought of before. All five of them had a good laugh at me. Huxley was the most searing in his comments on the impossibility of my ambition. His perspective came from the understanding that there is nothing new under the sun in psychotherapy, or possibly even in other areas of human thought. Anything you can think of, someone else has already thought of. Our task is not progress or development. Technology develops, but ethics, politics and psychotherapy don't. Our task is to give new forms to old wisdom, to unchanging and eternal ideas, making them relevant, attractive and interesting to the contemporary generations. So, we have to make up new similes, new metaphors, new songs, new tales; we have to discover new forms and new mediums. This is the role of creativity; this is where it's needed at the present moment. How can we convey the real and unchanging perennial truths most effectively right now, at this moment in time?

The best medicine, for me, against depression, melancholy and hopelessness is to honestly and bravely state what I believe in. Laing's purpose in his book *Wisdom, Madness and Folly*, or John Fowles' in *The Aristos* – both are "Credos", actually – is not to gain followers for their beliefs, but to inspire their readers to express and articulate their own credos. I have the same purpose in writing this book. Recently, after one of my lectures, a young woman in the audience was asked how she liked the talk. She had never heard me speak before and, to my surprise, she jokingly called me a stand-up philosopher. This really made me think, and gave me inspiration and motivation. Her opinion was the final nail in the coffin of my youthful ambition to impart knowledge. At the age of 70, I embarked on my new career as a performance artist.

At the beginning of the book, in the chapter "Ruptures", I write about seven great changes because I feel these changes characterise my life. A series of quick, cataclysmic changes or ruptures: something suddenly ends and something completely different gets under way. Recently, I reflected on how I am usually very quick to leave a situation, and I immediately enter another one. This is how I say my goodbyes as well. A break, a rupture, like quick scene changes in theatre. This is an aspect of my considerable resilience, for which I am grateful.

The chapter "Origins" introduces my philosophical ancestors. My aim here is not to impart information, but to invite interested readers to look up those I mention. The chapter is very short, only pointing out connections like a finger that points at the Moon. If you are interested in the Moon, don't try to suck the finger, go and discover the Moon for yourself.

As I was preparing to write *Credo*, I took out the journal I kept in London in 1974–75. I have returned to this material before, several times. I am grateful to past-Andrew for sensing that he was preparing a crucial gift for present-Andrew. Again, it was all new back then, all different, everything sparkling and surprising. Many times, I felt overwhelmed by the rapid phrasing, concepts, ideas and emotions. Even today, I often find that something emerges from between the lines, something that I've not seen or understood before. *Credo* is also a gift, I hope, to future-Andrew, so that he doesn't have to regret, on his death-bed, that he didn't pass on what he has received. As I was reading, I took notes, and I have now added the notes to the stories of those days.

I talk about Ronnie Laing a lot. One separate chapter and entire paragraphs here and there are dedicated to him. He appears a lot in the book because I had so many personal experiences with him, and I received so much defining intellectual inspiration from him. He would have been 90 years old in 2017, if he were still alive. In the summer of 1970, a few weeks before the birth of my son, I read his book *The Politics of Experience*, and I had a sudden realisation that the person who wrote the book knew me deeply and had the courage to say things I already knew and suspected but had not found the words to express. Maybe because I was scared? When I looked in his eyes, in 1974, I knew he was the first genius I had met. He could penetrate things down to their roots and see them for what they were. He didn't accept dogmas, and he took his own experiences seriously. He fought for freedom, he bravely looked into the soul of humanity, he was terrified of evil and he savoured the wonders of love and compassion.

In the chapter "Fantasy and Reality", I speculate about terms that don't really mean anything to me, like "self-knowledge", "self-development", and so on. For me, thinking and conjecturing have always been erotic experiences. Using pure logic to question the conceptual frameworks that we have been hypnotised to accept is a magnificent and terrifying game. This is what makes most people angry at me. This chapter might, hopefully, be an inspiration for many of my readers to be more daring in questioning the concepts of their own worlds, concepts that seem evident to everyone but don't actually mean anything at all. I also write about the real things that are fundamental elements of my credo, even if I have already discussed them in my other books. So, I write about the nature of responsibility and ethics, about freedom, individuality, community, solidarity, will and relationships. The latter, being an enormous topic deserving its own book, will be *The Book of Relationships,* the second volume of *A Guide for Lost Wanderers*, which I co-authored with Dorka Büky.

Credo is not an autobiography, although it contains many autobiographical elements; I didn't, however, worry about chronological order and definitely didn't bother to include everything. My hope is that, through the magnified moments in the book, readers will sense or see why I think the way I do: what I have lived through, the kind of experiences I had, what I saw, heard, read, what surprised and amazed me, what made me cry, what made me laugh, all the journeys I took on meandering detours until I arrived to where I am now. I have no intention of convincing anyone of anything. I just jotted down a few things I happened to come across.

I don't like to write. This book is a courageous endeavour. I have to be on my own to become absorbed in it. It is much more pleasant to talk with my patients or to give a presentation because this is how I can express my message: in company. My mind is quiet, and I rarely deliberate. When someone prods me to speak, I also listen in surprise to my own words. In Vancouver, I spend most of my time and energy with patients. Discussions are in English. I have this sense that, during therapy sessions, I breathe in and then, in Hungary, I breathe out.

English in, Hungarian out. Inhaling, exhaling. To me, somehow, it makes more sense to translate the Hungarian into English than the other way around. It might be because my mother tongue is Hungarian, and for my first years away from Hungary, I thought in Hungarian then translated my message into English. Now, I think in whichever language I use: Hungarian when I am with Hungarians, English when I am with English speakers. Now, I picture the reader and have a chat with them. I was 16 when I left Hungary, and I have been refining my Hungarian to the best of my ability since then. I translated Géza Gárdonyi's *Slave of the Huns*, and I have done several presentations and workshops in Hungarian. I am not afraid to use Hungarian, and I like the language even though my higher education was in English, and I have been dreaming in English for a long time. I hope my courage or boldness will inspire others to write down, to the best of their ability, what they believe in, which bright star guides their life and practice.

I have two projects in Hungary: the Feldmár Institute and the Soteria Foundation. I hope both will survive me. I wish that the spirit that guides me will strengthen them, so it will become obvious to everyone that love and compassion make our lives not just sustainable, but actually enjoyable. There is nothing else. Before I die, I'd like to sing, dance, play and work with a fervour that makes me forget myself.

RUPTURES

The Seventh One by Attila József[1]

Once you set foot on this earth,
Your mother gives you seven births!
Once in a blazing house afire,
Once in an icy flood's cold mire,
Once inside a loony bin,
Once amidst waving wheat so thin,
Once in cloister's hollow eye,
Once among pigs in the sty.
All six cry, it's not enough, son,
Be yourself the seventh one!

If an enemy stands before you,
Have seven men who'd stand up for you.
One who begins his day at leisure,
One who works his daily measure,
One who teaches gratis at his whim,
One who's thrown in the water to swim,
One who's the seed of a forest's growth of years,
One who's protected by his ancestor's tears.
But ruse or reproach won't get it done, –
Be yourself the seventh one!

If you'd go looking for a lover,
Have seven men try to find her.
One who for her word gives up his heart,
One who pays for his own part,
One who pretends to be a dreamer,

One who gropes her skirt to get her,
One who knows where her hooks can be found,
One who steps on her hanky on the ground, –
They all buzz like flies around carrion!
Be yourself the seventh one!

If you could afford to compile a tome,
Have seven men compose this poem.
One who builds a marble town,
One born asleep, his eyelids down,
One who charts the sky and knows it well,
One whose words can cast a spell,
One who sells his soul, trying to thrive,
One who carves up a rat while it's alive.
Two are brave and four are wise, son –
Be yourself the seventh one!

And if all this happened as was written,
Go to the grave as if you were all seven.
One who rocks on a milky chest,
One who grasps at dried hard breasts,
One who tosses away empty pans,
One who lends the poor his helping hands,
One who works like a man possessed,
One who stares at the Moon, obsessed;
You're already underground, my son!
Be yourself the seventh one!

I had a discussion, once, with Leon Redler and Ronnie Laing, about the possible origins of our suffering. The source of our pain might go back seven generations; one generation automatically, subconsciously, passes it on to the next. We are bound up in multigenerational curses. This poem, "The Seventh One", seems to encourage me to leave all this behind, to wake up and be myself, despite all reasons to the contrary. It also occurred to me that we all live on top of bloody mountains of corpses. Our ancestors sacrificed themselves, by the thousands, in battle for us to be born. Still, we have to relax and dissolve ourselves, if possible, from survival to living.

Each therapy session is a rupture. If I work for ten hours, that's ten ruptures. Surviving them taught me the resilience to quickly regain my own shape, despite each patient deforming me by impacting me. I don't remain stuck. This is some kind of elasticity, but I have to find words to discuss with the patient how they are trying to mould me because if they are trying to mould me, they are doing that to others as well. And if it's not good for me, it's not good for others.

First Rupture

The first rupture is me appearing from nothingness into something. Around 1938, my mother lived in a building on Tímár Street in Old Buda. She was twenty-something, and one day, she met my father on the common stairs. My father was a 38-year-old widower with no children. He started courting my mother and wasted no time getting to the point: did she want to have a family, because he wanted a child. So, by 1939, my mother was pregnant, but she miscarried the first baby. My father told her that if she didn't give birth to a child within a year, he would leave her. When she became pregnant again, the doctor recommended six months of bed rest. My mother stayed in bed and my father served her hand and foot. She ate a lot of sausages and pickled cucumbers, and didn't do much of anything. When I was born, on the 28th of October, 1940, my mother handed me to my father and told him. "Here is your son. Look after him." So, my father changed my nappies and fed me. My mother was running about because she got bored sick with all the lying down. I am not sure if she breastfed me at all. If she did, it was just for a very short time.

This is how I appeared in the world.

My Father

According to my mother, my father loved me like a mother. He accepted everything. In his eyes, everything was good. I could do nothing wrong. So, my mother had to play the role of the father. "Your father was morally insane," she said. "He used to smoke cigars and slurp his coffee." I associate these smells with my father. When I came home from school and got in the lift, the smell of cigars and sweet pastry in the air told me my father was home. He always brought me cakes. For a while, I had otitis media in both ears, every winter. The pain was terrible, and when the doctor was called, my father would sit me on his lap while the doctor stuck a needle through my eardrums to release the pus. When I broke my arm in the Mátra mountains, he was the one to come up and take me to Gyöngyös to the hospital. I could always rely on him. He was a quiet man. He didn't speak much.

After the war, when I was living with my mother and grandmother, I spent every Saturday afternoon from 12 to 2–3 o'clock at his place. I often pondered how I had so much to talk about with my mother and grandmother, even though we were constantly together. But with my father, it was as if we had nothing to say to each other, even though we hardly saw one another. Then my father bought a chess set, so we didn't just sit there in silence. We started playing chess, but it was still silent. Sometimes he fell asleep. He worked five and a half days every week, and he worked until midday on Saturday. He was tired, so he dozed off. When he took me to the opera, he nodded off sitting next to me. It felt awkward. I don't know if it was me who felt annoyed or if, when I told my mother, it was she who became indignant. With some of my memories, I am unsure if they are actually mine or come from my mother's commentary.

When I was about eight, my father took me to some conference on a train. We went to some place around Miskolc. It was not something that happened very often. I had a bowl of bouillon in the dining car, and I am still searching for its delightfully elusive taste. Even today, I would be so happy if I could find it. I've never had anything so delicious ever again. There was a party where we went, and with my height, my eyes were at the level of the grown-ups' hips. I felt relaxed. I didn't hold my father's hand. There were a lot of interesting women there, and I really liked one of them. I was madly attracted to her. She was dancing, and I grabbed her and buried my head, my face, into her arse. The woman turned around, picked me up and sat me on her lap. Then I saw her awesome breasts, so I buried my head into her bosom. It occurred to me, later on, that this woman must have been my father's lover. It may be that a child yearns for what his father likes. During the same trip, my father fell asleep in the hotel room with his cock hanging out. It seemed huge to me. It appeared almost a metre long compared to mine, and I pondered how mine would never get that big. I had never discussed this with my father. Once he had told me, although I didn't ask, how they used to compete as young men, trying to work out whose cock was longest. I was a mathematician, so I asked him how they measured it. "From the anus to the tip of the cock," he said. "With an erection, of course, because you have to measure the hard cock." These are the things one doesn't talk about in female company.

When he came, after me, to Toronto, Canada in 1959, I had just finished 13th grade and was about to graduate. During the end-of-the-year ceremony, I had to go up on stage to be presented with a small statue because, in the entire district, I had the best results in algebra, geometry, trigonometry, physics and chemistry. When I was presented with the award, there was a little speech about how this was a miracle because I had only been there for a year and hardly spoke English. I heard some loud sobs in the audience. It turned out to be my father, and I felt embarrassed. Later, when he was ill and dying, he called me over and asked me to lean in with my ear to his mouth. "Sarah thinks I am impotent, but that's only with her," he whispered, winking at me. Sarah was my father's wife. She was the nurse he met and fell in love with while in forced labour under the Nazis. "As you get older, make sure you are famous or rich, otherwise interesting women won't sleep with you." That was the only paternal advice he ever gave me, but I was already 32, not a child. He was a quiet man. He only spoke when he occasionally lost his temper. According to my mother, when someone told him the truth, that's when he'd hit the roof.

Second Rupture

In early 1944, the Nazis took my father for forced labour, and put my grandmother in the ghetto. After that, it was just the two of us, my mother and I, on Kis Rókus Street, in Buda, the area of Budapest to the west of the Danube. By that time, all hell had broken loose. Somehow, I have this impression that my mother knew they would come for us, as well, but instead of trying to escape, she waited. Later, around the time I was 50 years old, a very intense memory surfaced. It gave me a terrible, unstoppable shaking/shivering episode. She didn't just wait. She wanted to kill me and then kill herself, but she couldn't bring herself to do it. One day, there was a knock on the door and an Arrow Cross man asked whether or not she was Erzsébet Feldmár, because he was going to take us to the internment jail right away. Somehow, my mother managed to talk him around, and he let her leave me with the building janitor. That's when we said goodbye. I was only three and half years old and had no idea what was going on. The janitor sent me to play in the courtyard. There was a huge puddle there. I walked around it several times, but I was a good boy, so I didn't step in it. I don't know who, whether it was my mother or my father, and I don't know how, but someone got in touch with Irén Igaz, who came and picked me up. (In Hungarian, *igaz* means "righteous" and "true".) That was the beginning of a year-and-a-half-long rupture, when I lived with the Igaz family without my father, my mother or my grandmother.

We had to keep my identity a secret. We had to lie to everyone and say that my name was Andrew Igaz. Actually, I have no clear memories of this time. I used meditation, therapy, and hypnosis to try and regress to that time, when I was between the ages of three-and-a-half and five. It is as if there is an insurmountable wall protecting those memories. My soul ejected me, didn't let me enter. I remember a warm loving feeling that Irén's body, her presence, gave me. It was always good to nestle into her. When she was there with me, I wasn't scared.

Irén Igaz

Irén Igaz is important. Joseph Brodsky[2] once said, at an American university commencement, that nowadays it is impossible to avoid coming across evil. The more we try to avoid it, the more evil approaches us. But how should we behave when we come face to face with it? If it kills us, that's quite straightforward; but if we survive, then we want to remember this encounter without having to spit at ourselves in the face when we look in the mirror. Irén Igaz told me the exact same thing when, decades later, she described something that happened while I stayed with them. One day, an Arrow Cross man knocked on her door and informed her that he knew she was hiding a Jewish child. Irén begged him to spare the child. The man replied that if Irén slept with him, he would let her off and not take the child. She asked for a day to think about it. She thought about her husband, who was in a forced-labour battalion. She thought about how people can't just sleep with her. She thought about how she couldn't be certain whether the Arrow Cross man would keep his word and really spare the child, even if she slept with him. But she didn't really think about all that because she knew if she didn't sleep with the man, and I was taken away, she could never look into a mirror ever again. The Arrow Cross man wasn't extraordinarily vicious, so he kept his word. Once he got what he wanted, he let me alone and let me live.

The mirror test is important. According to Joan Halifax[3], the most dangerous addiction is not heroin or cocaine, but life. In Buddhist practice, one must give up attachment even to life itself. Sometimes we have to give up what we are dependent on: propriety, morality, principles, faith, loyalty, alcohol and sometimes even life itself. If we are dependent on something, if we are addicted to life, it is easier to become victims of evil, and it is easier to become evil.

Third Rupture

A year and a half later, near the end of 1945, just after my fifth birthday, my father, who had returned from forced labour with

Sarah and taken me back 4–5 months previously, told me I had a belated birthday present waiting for me. I was overjoyed because I really wanted a big wooden truck at the time, and I didn't get one for my birthday. When my father said I would be getting something after all, I thought, yippee! The truck is coming! We went somewhere, and there were crowds of people sitting and standing all over the place. My father crouched down next to me and pointed at a woman, saying, "Look, that's your mother!" My mother had been rounded up and deported to Auschwitz in March, 1944. She returned in early November, 1945. She survived because she was young, strong and could speak German fluently. The Germans used her as a labourer in a dynamite factory. I didn't have the faintest idea who this woman was. I didn't recognise her. I remember feeling seriously deceived and disappointed. "Who is this woman, and where is my truck?" I thought. I remember feeling averse to her, but I don't have any visual memories of what happened. I don't remember her face; I only remember these feelings. Later on, I found out that a child of three and a half can only keep their mother alive in their soul for a certain period of time. By that time, my mother had died in my soul. They told me she was my mother, but I didn't *know* her as my mother, and I think it was difficult to believe anyway.

But I do have some vague memories of going for a walk with my actual mother on our first day together, after she returned. I was holding her hand and said, "Sarah is very beautiful, but you are a lot more beautiful." She asked who Sarah was, and I told her she was my father's girlfriend. There was a big row between my parents that day, and although my father kept promising that he would get rid of ("liquidate" was the word he used) Sarah, my mother still kicked him out. Somehow, she was jealous of Irén as well, and she forbade me from seeing her again. As for the reason, I am not sure whether she was worried that I loved Irén more than her, that I had somehow become hers, or she may have figured out that Irén was one of my father's lovers (to this day, I am unsure whether she was or she wasn't). I don't know which one is true. But for me, this created another rupture. Later, as an adult, I had this recurring dream of walking on the tarmac of a big open-air carpark and a truck is driving towards me. It hits me. Its metal grill smashes into me and sends me flying into the air. When I stop flying, I start hurtling down and crash into the tarmac. I am hit in the chest twice: once leaving the earth and once meeting the earth again. Separation and reintegration were both huge and painful events.

My Mother

My mother was proud of her legs, and she used to show them off whenever she had the chance. Her face and eyes looked like she was always suspicious, as if she was squinting. She was a heavy smoker, and smoked at least a pack a day. The smoke also made her squint. For a long time, I had this feeling that she could see inside me. I needed a lot of courage to start lying to her. When she hugged me, she squeezed me very tightly. I couldn't cuddle up to her; she grabbed me and pulled me in, then pushed me away. Sometimes, when she was asleep, I could nestle into her. She was brave and had no respect for those she considered cowards. Apparently, she was the first woman to go rowing on the Danube. She liked to sunbathe. When she was doing chores around the house, I had to hide, because if she saw me reading, she would snap at me for not helping. She was often angry, and then I had to appease her. I couldn't fall asleep until she forgave me. She was quick to anger. She occasionally chased her mother, my grandmother, around the table with a knife.

In the summer, we used to go to the Mátra mountains for a few months. I was free to roam there. We had an agreement, my mother and I, that I could go and play with the other kids, but as soon as I heard her whistle, I had to go home straight away. It was a small village, and she could whistle very loudly. Once, in the middle of some amazing game, I heard her whistle. I left everything and ran straight home, only to see her chatting with the woman next door. When I arrived, panting, she turned to her and said, "See, if I whistle, he comes." What usually started our arguments was her almost hypnotic suggestions that I had to obey her. "Andrew, are you deaf?!?!" she used to scream, if I didn't obey. The implication being that, if I had heard her, I should have done what she wanted. She treated me as if I were her puppet. When I wasn't how she wanted me to be, she asked me, "Where is my Andrew? Where did this boy come from? My Andrew would have never said this, he would have never done this." She laid this guilt trip on me that I was driving her insane, and she was going to end up in a loony bin because of me. She also often told me that I had to do what she said because she only survived for me, she only came back because of me. If I didn't exist, she could have died peacefully, but for me she survived, she came home, and I can't even be bothered to take out the rubbish.

I was 15 when I fell in love with Olga, who was a year older. I was really in love. My mother saw Olga somewhere once, and from then on, she was always going on about "how could you possibly fall in love with such an ugly, plain-looking girl?". And she didn't know that Olga was Catholic, I didn't dare tell her. That was the time I realised I had to lie to her. Anything I told her would be used against me. My mother was my constant headwind, always growing stronger and stronger until I could hardly move. She was always against me, never next to me or behind me. She would always say that I was so desperately ugly and intolerable, there was no woman on earth who could put up with me. She was the only one in this whole wide world who could tolerate me. But it wasn't because she liked me. Oh, no. It was that being my biological mother meant she had no choice. She said I shouldn't even dream about someone liking me because I didn't deserve it. I tried to stand up for myself, but it was impossible. I learned to stay quiet because each word added fuel to the fire. This infuriated her even more, and in her fierce, seething rage, she would turn away from me, enveloping herself in a wounded silence. I was dependent on that relationship.

As I sat on the train later that year, in 1956, travelling towards the border, I felt a distinct sense of wanting to be caught and taken back. I was scared of the future, of being on my own. Yet, even by the age of ten, I had a clear understanding that it was difficult to live with her. I even discussed it with my grandmother. Actually, it was my grandmother who saved me from derangement because she was my accomplice against my mother. I also spoke with my father, once, about how living with my mother was pure hell. I was maybe 16 years old, and I asked him why he had left me. He said it was difficult living with my mother. "But if you knew that, why did you leave me with her?" I asked. "Because of the law and because everybody was of the opinion that a small child is better off with their mother," he said. "Well, fuck that!" I replied. At least I could give him a piece of my mind.

I don't think my mother would have ever sought help from a psychotherapist. She was completely independent. She didn't respect anyone and didn't take anyone seriously. She was thoroughly convinced that no one in existence understood her. She told me I was terrible for loving Olga because she didn't want any woman to take me away from her. She was jealous of everyone. Despite constantly finding faults with me, she used to boast about me to others. Behind my back, she used to say positive things about me, but never to my face. Whenever I work with a family that includes a parent like her, I encourage the child to run away. After all, that is how my father interceded on my behalf, shortly after my sixteenth birthday. When he brought up his idea, that this was the last chance to leave the country, he opened the door of my cage. It wasn't easy because I was still young, and he didn't say he would come with me. But I respect him for opening the cage and helping me escape.

I was scared on the train. I wasn't in the least eager to go, but I still managed to escape somehow. I used to write long letters to my parents from London and then from Toronto, and that brought my mother and father closer together again. Whenever I wrote to one of them, he or she would share it with the other, and they would meet up to read my letters. A few years later, they all joined me: my mother, my father and Sarah, his wife. So, I ended up living under the same roof with my mother once more, who hadn't changed at all. In fact, she had become worse. I was in love with Mary at the time. She visited, and I locked the door of my room from the inside. My mother started knocking, then banging on the door, and she screamed that the whore had to leave that minute. I moved away after that, as I was almost 20, and spent less and less time with my mother from then on. But to this very day, I am scared of women's wrath. It is possible that I subconsciously recreate the situations I am used to because I quite often manage to infuriate women, even now. My mother never allowed herself to be sad. She turned her sadness into rage. Anger gives you a backbone. She was terrified of sadness, and I may be more scared of a woman being sad than her being angry. Maybe I would have been most terrified if I saw my mother crying and losing it. But she didn't cry, she screamed. She preferred blowing up to breaking down.

Fourth Rupture

In 1956, when I was in year 11 in high school, I was in love with Olga. I used to argue with my mother all the time. I got bad grades in Russian, I hated geography and history, I was scared I would fail my exams, and I wouldn't be able to go to university because my father wasn't loyal enough to the regime. And then, all of a sudden, we got sent home from school, from Rákóczi Gymnasium because, apparently, the revolution had broken out.

It was the 23rd of October. The 28th was my birthday, my sixteenth. We all lived in the basement cellar for a while, where we were in full earshot of each other's lives. We could hear everything from lovemaking to quarrels. Every so often, I had to run up to the apartment on the fourth floor to get this or that. I remember looking out towards Széna Square through the cracked, broken glass in the window and seeing Russian tanks rolling along Margit Boulevard towards us. On one of them, the gun turret started to turn slowly and I was frozen by a sudden, enormous blast, by bright flames and a whistling sound as the tank shot a huge missile straight towards me. At least that's how it seemed to me. The missile smashed into the house next door, but I still nearly shat my pants. I raced downstairs to the cellar. Sometimes, when we needed bread, I was sent to the bakery. I had to dash across Margit Boulevard, and at the bakery, people were standing in line, as close to the wall as possible. Once, one of my classmates arrived just after me, and we were chatting away when a tank rolled onto the street. As it hurtled past us, its machine gun opened fire, throwing flames and bullets. Every second person in the line collapsed on the floor. They were either dead or injured. At that moment, my classmate died next to me.

Despite the unpredictability of the fighting, my mother sometimes went over to Pest to work. She was a seamstress and was expected to keep her deadlines. I went to pick her up in the afternoons because I was worried about her. There was no public transport, no buses and no trams. I hitched rides, holding onto the back of lorries, and that's how I reached her. There was a stretch of road I had to walk along. Once, I had to jump over strange, two-foot-long, coal-black, doll-like things. Someone was examining one of them, so I asked him what they were. He said they were charred Russian soldiers. They got stuck in their tank when a Molotov cocktail engulfed them in flames. They baked to coal inside and, when the tank blew up, they were thrown all over the place.

My father used to live on Kossuth Square, near the Parliament. A tank was parked on the tracks of Tramline 2. There were Russian soldiers sitting on the tank. They were eating, drinking and chatting with each other. I was with a few high-school friends, and we approached the soldiers. We spoke enough Russian to ask them what they were doing here. They didn't even know where they were. They were Armenians, thinking they had been deployed at the Suez. There was a Ukrainian soldier among them, and he said if this was Budapest, they would get out, they wouldn't fight. Then there was a sudden ringing noise and they swiftly climbed into the tank, pulled the roof over, and as they disappeared, they shouted at us to clear off because they just got orders to shoot. We ran into my father's house, and there was shooting outside for hours.

Then, the day before Christmas, when I visited my father, he asked if I wanted to see the world and study at a Western university. The borders were still somewhat open, and although the Russians had already quashed the revolution, he had a contact, a farmer, who could take me over the border for some money. I told him I would think about it, but by the next day, I knew I would go. I don't know where I got this decision from, I just knew that if I went, I wouldn't have to go to school any more, I wouldn't have to learn Russian and, especially, I wouldn't have to argue with my mother ever again. I was scared, but I said yes. My mother, of course, accused my father of conspiring to take her son away. A few days before New Year's Eve, I left for the border. At that point, if someone was caught at the border, they noted their name down, but didn't hurt them. So, throughout my journey, I was hoping to get caught. But it wasn't to be. That day, maybe two out of a hundred people got through, and I was one of those two. After a long and arduous journey, I got to Toronto, where a completely new life began with my aunt and uncle.

Fifth Rupture

About three or four years after my parents turned up in Toronto, and I was back living with my mom, I moved with my soon-to-be wife Mary down to Baltimore, Maryland. I had received a scholarship in math and theoretical statistics from Johns Hopkins University, which had the crucial advantage of not having to live in the same city as my mother. That was my first escape from Toronto. My tenure in Baltimore and my marriage to Mary both came to an untimely end. She cheated on me with my best friend, we got a divorce, and I fell apart.

I moved back to Toronto and started working for the Imperial Oil company (Esso) as a mathematician, and IT and coding specialist. I also started psychoanalysis because I felt that life and I were both hopeless. I felt cut off from everyone and everything. I couldn't pay attention to anything, I couldn't be happy about anything, and I didn't feel like doing anything. I spoke with the head of psychiatry at Johns Hopkins University, and he recommended a psychoanalyst who told me that the magnitude of my emotions was evidence that my past had invaded my present. So, we needed to examine my old traumas to see which ones were undigested. The analysis lasted nine months. I had five sessions every week. Imperial Oil had an excellent medical insurance policy, so when I included the expenses of psychoanalysis in my tax returns, I was awarded so much tax credit, I even made some money. Psychoanalysis could be written off as a medical expense because I was "ill". The benefit of going to five sessions a week was the discussions had so much depth. Much later, I ended up with two patients, myself, who came to see me just as often. When one has therapy that often, one quickly realises one should talk about how one feels, not about what was happening in one's life. When there is no story, one finds that one has to express "what is" in a spontaneous and honest way. One shouldn't hide things or feel ashamed with the therapist. Well, as a result of my long therapy, I realised I could be a better therapist than my analyst.

A few years later, in 1967, I saw an ad for a job at Western Ontario University in London, Ontario. An IT professor was looking for a developer who was interested in learning psychology because they had a project to develop a programme for psychiatric interviews. I called and went to see him. His name was Zenon Pylyshyn, and he gave me the job right away. Pylyshyn also got me into the psychology department, and my MA in Psycholinguistics began. I was working and studying. Around this time, I met Meredith, whom I later married. When I completed my MA in 1969, I received an invitation for a two-month summer fellowship in psycholinguistics from a professor in Vancouver, British Columbia. I immediately accepted. Vancouver was at the other end of the continent from Toronto, and I fell in love with it as soon as I arrived. I never wanted to return to Toronto ever again.

Sixth Rupture

It wasn't easy, however, to settle in Vancouver. After the two-month fellowship ended in August of 1969, and after returning to London, Ontario, I moved to Urbana-Champaign, which is a couple of hours south of Chicago, to attend the University of Illinois for my PhD. I started work on my degree with Charles E. Osgood. My plan was to get my PhD in psycholinguistics and then move to Vancouver. The university was set among cornfields; as far as the eye could see, there was a flat sea of corn. I was sitting in the middle of all this, working with huge computers, developing programmes, and feeling bored out of my mind. My relationship with Meredith was progressing at this time, however, and I decided to leave the university and not stay just for the sake of a PhD. So, I took my leave of Osgood, who was very kind and understanding, just like a good father. He asked me if I needed some money and offered some from his own pocket. He was very different from my supervisor at Johns Hopkins, who was livid when I quit. He got really angry at me for abandoning the scholarship he went out of his way to get for me. Hence, I should fuck off. But Osgood was very decent.

Meredith and I drove to Vancouver, then, in the early fall of 1969, and I started looking for work there as a clinical psychologist because I didn't want to have anything to do with psycholinguistics anymore. I got a job with the government of British Columbia straight away. I started working in a mental health centre with three others: a psychiatrist, a psychiatric social worker and a mental health nurse. The psychiatrist came from England, had an English accent, and when I told him I had no experience whatsoever, he said the same thing as Ronnie Laing told me later on. It's better to know nothing than to have your head full of damaging, useless misconceptions. He suggested I could work with the children because the children are honest, guileless, and they would teach me everything. "You can't learn from adults," he said. So that's how I started working in the field. I read the book *Dibs in Search of Self*, in which author and psychologist Virginia Axline describes her therapy with a child named Dibs. I learned everything I needed to start. I set up a table full of sand and another table with water. I placed loads of little toys all around, including horses, pigs and hand puppets. All sorts of people and their children started coming. That's how I began my new life. It was brilliant. The psychiatrist worked with the fathers, the social worker with the mothers, the nurse with the older children, and I worked with the little ones.

Seventh Rupture

I had worked as a psychotherapist for five years before I went to see R.D. Laing in London. That was how the boy become a man, how I gained the respect of someone I respected, and how I started to become a real healer. I wasn't born a healer, after all; I had to learn it from someone who knew how to do it.

At the beginning of February 1975, about five months after I arrived in London, I started having a sense that everything had fallen apart. Everything I had known, or thought I knew, became invalid, and it became apparent that I wouldn't be able to continue with my work as before. I had no idea how I could/would continue.

I felt completely lost, I plunged into the depths, I became desperate and I felt very depressed. I wasn't even sure if I could earn enough money to stay in London with my family. I felt unable to do anything. This nosedive lasted about a month, and when I started making more money, that pulled me out of it. I worked as a math tutor and advertised my services as a hypnotist in *Time Out* magazine. In Vancouver, since 1970, I had visited every dentist, psychologist and psychiatrist who used hypnosis. I asked them all to hypnotise me and teach me how to do it. I wanted to learn what it could be used for. I had read every book available on the subject, especially the ones by Milton H. Erickson. Paul Bakan, who had worked in Ernest Hilgard's Stanford Laboratory of Hypnosis Research, was one of my professors at Simon Fraser University.

More and more people came for hypnosis, and the idea of it even attracted those who would otherwise have never gone to therapy. Having money was a huge help, and everyone who came gave me more experience with people. Working hard helped me overcome the crisis. Laing encouraged me, and he told me that despondency was to be expected. It was not at all surprising. If someone is taught to play the piano when they are young, but they have a faulty technique and use the wrong fingers, it is much harder for them to relearn the piano with a good music teacher than it is for a person who has no prior experience at all. The one with the poor technique has to give up using the wrong fingers and has to get used to something completely different. By considering the crisis to be a transformation of habits, Laing normalised the situation for me and everything became a lot easier. I could deal with it, and I didn't have to be ashamed and impatient. Up to that point, I thought it was difficult because

I was a moron, which is what my mother used to say. Then Laing told me the reason I found it difficult was because it was difficult. Well, as a child, I had never been told anything like that.

Laing

In 1973, I had begun the PhD programme in clinical psychology at Simon Fraser University. In February of 1974, Laing arrived in Vancouver, towards the end of his North American tour. In January of that year, Erich Fromm had also visited the city. They were my favourite thinkers at that time. I got to know them both, and had some discussions with each of them. Within ten minutes of meeting Fromm, I knew I was going to read his books, but I didn't want to work with him. He exuded a sense of precision and chilliness. I felt no personal attraction to him. At that point, I had been working as a psychologist with children and families for almost five years, and I was going through a crisis. I was worried I wasn't doing things properly, but I couldn't find a teacher I wanted to work with. To put it more precisely, I wasn't even sure what was happening. Was I doing well but unable to believe it, in which case I needed therapy; or was I really not doing things properly, in which case I needed a teacher and apprenticeship? Laing held a seminar for psychotherapists in Vancouver during his visit. There were maybe forty of us, and the first question he put to us was whether we were genuine healers or had we found a great ego trip as therapists where we can always triumph over our patients. The question cut me to the core. I had to decide which one I was. Was this just an ego trip or was I a healer? During the break, I asked Laing how I could recognise if I was a healer. He told me that either you were born one, or you became one by being an apprentice of a healer. I didn't think for even a second before asking him if I could be his apprentice. He told me his practice was in London, England, but if I could be there, something would surely happen in this regard. If not with him, then with someone from his circle.

By September 1974, I was in London. Laing himself accepted me into therapy and supervised me as a therapist. For one year, I spent about seven hours with him every week. Not long before we had met, Laing lived in Sri Lanka for a year, where he spent most of his time meditating. He told me how he used to have his office on Harley Street, and just like all the other psychiatrists, he received his patients wearing a suit and tie and well-polished shoes. After he had been in India and Sri Lanka, he started working from home, barefoot, sitting cross-legged and without a tie. He was surprised by the significant change in the kind of people who came to see him. He never considered himself a rock star or a revolutionist. He wasn't a follower or member of any "ism" or school of thought, and he was surprised when he became world-famous after his book *The Politics of Experience* was published. It had never occurred to him that millions of people would relate to what he described. After Kingsley Hall, the first Laingian asylum, there were seven shelters dotted around London under the umbrella of the Philadelphia Association, of which Laing was a founding member. Only the venue changed. The project and the experiment continued.

After my arrival, I started going to two of these shelters right away. Laing was a genius who had read all the books in Glasgow's great central library by the time he was 16. He was very familiar with the history of European thought, and was well-acquainted with medical science, psychiatry and philosophy. He was the first person, for instance, to present French philosopher Jean-Paul Sartre in English-speaking countries. I'll never forget sitting on the sofa with him for hours, reading a book by French psychoanalyst Jacques Lacan. He called this a "close" reading. We read slowly, carefully, analysing each sentence. We finished three pages in four hours. He was brave, honest and spontaneous. A dangerous man, who was always immediately prepared to say whatever he thought. He didn't have time for false, pretentious people. He never gave in to any social convention. He ate his dinner standing up and fell asleep when he was bored, even if he happened to be in the middle of holding a group session. There were many who misunderstood him – maybe because if you took him seriously and actually understood him, you had to change your life, or at least consider why you wouldn't.

There was some speculation about his ideas. Apparently, he considered the mothers, parents or families of schizophrenic people responsible for that person's "illness". This is a barefaced lie. He was of the opinion that, to become schizophrenic, to exhibit those symptoms, one needed a certain genetic disposition. It is inherited and may be genetically predetermined, but such a disposition in itself is not sufficient for the thing to develop. For the person to become a "successful case", they would also need a certain environment. It is like musical talent, according to Laing. We wouldn't know Mozart if he hadn't been exceptionally talented genetically *and* lived in a very musical household. His father played music every day, taught him and made him practise from a very young age. If these circumstances hadn't been present, it is possible that Mozart would have become a cobbler, whistling away enthusiastically while repairing shoes. On more than one occasion, Laing told his "ambitious" patients that he could see them yearning to go mad, but they were bound to fail because they lacked any modicum of talent. Gregory Bateson[4] was the first to speak about the "double bind". This happens when a mother is ambivalent with her child. She calls them to her with one hand and pushes them away with the other. The child becomes paralysed, frozen. The child gets angry because any move they make is the wrong move. This maddening situation, coupled with denying the role of the mother, produces within moments the disturbing, dangerous, frightened, and "schizophrenic" child.

Laing regarded himself as a doctor, primarily, and a psychiatrist, secondarily. He was guided by the Hippocratic oath first and foremost. The basic essence of this oath is to do no harm. Laing considered many of his colleagues "anti-psychiatrists", at least those who treated their patients inhumanely. They poisoned their patients with medications they themselves would never have taken. In other words, the anti-psychiatrists were the ones who harmed those who had asked for their help. The deeper essence of the Hippocratic oath is to not make the life of those who allowed the doctor to enter it more difficult and unpleasant than it would have been without the doctor. One who wants to improve others' lives, one who wants to help, is already treading the path to hell.

Thomas Szász[5], in his countless works, only really emphasises a few crucial ideas. One of these ideas is that mental illness doesn't exist. It is just a very bad metaphor. If you have brain problems, go and see a neurologist or a brain surgeon. But other problems don't really belong to the realm of medical science because they are produced by life's difficulties. Laing completely agreed with this idea. Szász was a libertarian. He fought for and defended every individual's freedom, including the freedom of lunatics. He deemed all force and forced treatment to be a criminal offence. After all, if a diabetic doesn't take their insulin, no one will call the police. What need is there to call the police if a so-called lunatic doesn't take their antipsychotic medication? One of Laing's objectives was to put an end to the use of force. He and Szász agreed on that. But Szász misunderstood Laing's practice. Laing believed that if mental illness doesn't exist, there was no need for a healer. Szász didn't understand that, in one of Laing's shelters, the residents were given complete freedom. The only rule was this: whatever is not forbidden is allowed. And it rested on the community of residents to decide what came to be forbidden. Laing's practice consisted of discussions and interactions without labels. He called this "interpersonal phenomenology, a branch of social phenomenology.

Laing didn't belong to any political factions, he didn't believe in any dogma, and everything was up for debate. His favourite question was "Are you sure about that?" He was deeply skeptical but never cynical. He criticised and tried to accept both the political right and left, but he was never committed to either of them. He was a deeply ethical person, like Emmanuel Levinas or Martin Buber, and he had a distinct perspective that a person is mad if they have dogmas because they will deem it acceptable to hurt another person in the name of an ideology. According to Szász, psychotherapy was Freudian, Jungian or some other psychoanalyst-ian. And a psychotherapist was someone who adhered to a particular school of thought. Szász noticed that Laing wasn't doing that. He was doing something different. Laing simply accepted solidarity with the patient and kept encouraging them until the patient became emancipated. Laing never criticised me – unlike my mother, who constantly criticised me – and, somehow, I managed to earn his respect. He could sense that I understood him when so many people misinterpreted him. I was eager to take advantage of any opportunity he gave me, and I never refused when he sent me to deal with a crisis. No matter how scared I was, I plunged right in. I chose my words carefully, I thought things over, and I wasn't afraid to ask questions. I respected him, I didn't ask for more than what he was giving, and I was careful not to overstep his boundaries. He was a person who finally showed a reflection of myself like no one ever had before. My father reflected an image that told me I was worthy of love, but I didn't respect him, so that image didn't matter. I only saw my father through the eyes of my mother. My mother saw him as a weak, sentimental man who was incapable of disciplining me. He was a useless waste of space, as far as she was concerned. So, I couldn't rely on my father's emotions. They didn't help.

But Laing was a formidable man. He was very strong, and if he liked me, I could believe I was actually worthy of love. Laing was affectionate, kind, and polite with me. He spoke to me as though I was more intelligent and educated than I thought I was. As a result of the year's intense work with him, I got up to the point he saw me at, from the very beginning. When I first went to see him in London, I felt I was a puny frog, but he magically transformed me into a proper prince. There was something erotic about my relationship with him, but never in a homosexual way. Eroticism is a very positive energy. When two people are delighted with each other, when they enjoy each other's strength, beauty, skill or dazzling intellect, either from far away or close up – that is eroticism. Men wrestling, women walking arm-in-arm, couples dancing: they all enjoy the magic of eroticism. This love doesn't have to open up towards the sexuality of genitals that yearns for orgasm. There is no need to be scared of that. Thinking, contemplating, speculating, and all the excitements of the mind are among the most erotic things in the world. Laing unlocked the world of men for me. For a long time, I was afraid of getting close to men and Laing helped me understand that there was no need to be scared of them. One can be delighted with them. It is intriguing that, in the beginning, 90 percent of my patients were women. At the age of 60, the proportion was 50–50, and nowadays, there are 60 percent men to 40 percent women. These changes may be a possible indication of my development as a therapist and as a person.

Once, Laing and I had a conflict. We were flying to Cortes Island on a small aircraft, and I was telling him about how my mother used to describe me as ugly and contemptible, and how pleased I was to be over this. That night on the island, he looked at me and he said, "Well, you know, just because your mother said you were ugly doesn't mean you are not ugly. Your mother was right. It is impossible for anyone to be attracted to you, even your wife is lying. She is painting beautiful pictures of you because she is afraid of painting the reality." First, I thought he was teasing me, and I was laughing along, but after half an hour, I started to feel quite uncomfortable. Yet he kept repeating the same thing. He didn't stop. I started believing him. "Well, fuck off then!" I screamed, walking out and slamming the door. The next morning, at breakfast, he grunted an apology. Maybe he went too far, he said. But anyway, it was definitely useful for one thing: I should never have thought I got over my mother because, if I had, he couldn't have provoked me to such pain and anger. I don't know if there was a justification for that. But one thing comes to mind. In his seminar, Francis Huxley spoke about George Ivanovitch Gurdjieff[6], who gave his students bizarre tasks: Go out in the garden and dig a deep hole, then fill it in and level it out; or, move and when he gives the sign, stand still. Once, trembling in fear, one of his students said, "No, leave me alone, I am not doing this any longer." Gurdjieff's eyes lit up, and he congratulated the student. Actually, I realised Laing had also wanted me to stand up for myself because when I could do that, the curse of what my mother said was lifted. A lot of therapists are of the opinion that they have to talk with the patient, pass on the knowledge. Laing believed one had to offer an experience to the other person. Well, he certainly provided me with an experience I'll never forget. But one thing is sure: I never treat my patients like that.

It is a paradox that he allowed himself to live and behave in ways that would disturb others, while he wanted those with power to accept and understand him. He knew it was a paradox. We once had to appear on a TV show in Vancouver, and I wore an open-neck shirt. He looked at me and told me to wear a tie. "What's going on?" I thought. "Is he trying to be my father?" He looked at me, and he said "If you look like a hippie, no one will ever take you seriously. If it is important that they take us seriously, then we shouldn't create obstacles that would make it more difficult for them to do so." Sometimes, that was what he wanted, and at other times, he didn't care. His mind warned him to be careful, but he also had resistance. It was like Penelope from the ancient Greek myths, who undid the weaving for the shroud she had woven during the day at night, so she wouldn't have to give herself to anyone. Laing always had this duality: half of him was bound to heaven, the other half to hell. The good and the bad fought in him. His desire, his dream, was to be accepted just as he was, without paying the price of having to behave well. I am more "acceptable" than he was. My temperament is different, yet his example still stirs me to monitor and curb any remnant of habits to appease others or compromise myself.

After Laing's death, at the memorial gathering, Phyllis Chesler[7] gave a talk about him. She referred to him as a true feminist who really paid attention to women and took them seriously. He liked the company of women, and he liked the company of men, too. He liked everything. He was a "polymorphous pervert". Still, there was something masculine about this whole Laing thing. The masculine is logos. We talk about what can be talked about, and we don't talk about what can't be talked about, and when we talk, we talk about things precisely. This is the masculine intellect; the masculine is a sword that says *this* is not *that*. There is no emotion in using a sword, there is nothing personal about it, you just need the appropriate skill. Laing never stated anything positively. He remained a skeptic to the very last particle of his being.

What was personal about him? He always spoke about his own conclusions and about his own experiences and thoughts. This is a crucial core principle of the work Laing and I did together, and for others. We didn't want to pass on dogmas; rather, we wanted to question everything. We inquired and speculated. This is hard for a lot of people. This approach can come across as ignorant to some people, and they themselves don't want to appear ignorant. Others miss something to hold on to, the fixed point, piece of knowledge, that can be the basis for understanding the world. There aren't many people who are brave enough to risk the independence of dogma-free existence. Truth be told, one must learn a lot to be able to let go of everything they have learned. The Philadelphia Association of London was formed as an alliance of five men. They had a loose, casual working relationship. Laing thought that if they were closer to each other, if the ties were stronger, that would create too much tension, and sooner or later, the whole thing would explode. So, there was distance, spaciousness, there was freedom, and no constraints, because masculine energy has a hard time tolerating others' differences. As soon as someone is different, that immediately generates the question or notion of trying to decide which one is better, which one is worse, and sooner or later they kill each other. So, these five men managed to get on with each other.

They each had their own kingdom, or their own autonomous shelter. Each shelter had its own characteristics, just as each man leading it had his own attributes. But they all agreed that none of them would know the only truth, none of them would know best or be most definite, so they agreed on having no dogmas. That was the only dogma. Everything that was not forbidden was allowed, so nothing was forbidden at first. The rules came about later, one after the other, in a different way, and at different times in each shelter, whenever and in whatever way they became necessary. If something came up, they had to discuss it. When John Heaton, for instance, became too close with one of his patients, and their relationship became too intimate, Laing held him accountable. And when Laing did something the others didn't like, then he was held accountable. Still, it was obvious to everyone that Laing was the *primus inter pares*.[8] He was the appeal. No matter how smart and great the others were, they didn't possess his charisma. A certain hierarchy evolved. Heaton felt he was equal to Laing. They grew up in the same current of thought, after all, and were twins, as it were. Leon Redler was the younger brother in this family. Most debates and discussions were about philosophy, ethics or politics. Politics, of course, not in the sense of which party to support, but in the Aristotelian sense of internal influence, power dynamics, and current organisational issues. There were some people, though not many, Laing looked up to, but he usually considered himself equal to everyone. He had an armchair, and if someone sat in it, he asked them to stand up and find another chair because that was his. As far as I know, he only offered that chair to anyone once: he offered it to Heinz Cassirer, who translated the New Testament from Greek into English.

In contemporary global intellectual thought, there aren't any thinkers like Laing, no defining intellects with landmark theories that turn everything upside down. He had an important position, and there have been no candidates since to fill his shoes. Anyone who has ever tried has been excommunicated, neglected, and/ or forgotten. Who has heard of Stanislav Grof, who developed a cartography of the human psyche?[9] Thomas Szász had already asserted that "mental illness" is an evil metaphor, but we still use it today, as if Szász had never existed. Laing is said to be "outdated", although we didn't pay attention to him even when we should have.

When he died, I received two of his books as presents: one by Ludwig Wittgenstein and one by Simone Weil.[10] Both authors are important to me. The first encourages me to formulate my thoughts clearly, and the second provokes me to speak about the spirit beyond the psyche.

ORIGINS

I have two families in terms of my intellectual history: the psychoanalytic and the philosophical. The psychoanalytic line, which itself has several sources, starts with the main line of Sigmund Freud. He was possibly the first doctor to genuinely pay attention to women and to take them seriously. He recognised that hysteria is not an illness but the struggle of the weak against the strong. After a public presentation of a man with hysteria, Freud was ridiculed at first. But he managed to prove that not just women, but some men, are also powerless, and this powerlessness results in them being labelled hysterical; it has nothing to do with their particular gender. His case studies are enjoyable to read. They are pure phenomenology, but his theories transform into dangerously rigid dogmas. This branch continues through Melanie Klein to D.W. Winnicott. Eric Graham Howe is a separate branch, as is Charles Rycroft.

Laing emerged from these three branches. He attended Winnicott's analysis and studied under his supervision. Laing also used to see and work with Rycroft, and his writings influenced Laing deeply. Their relationship ended when Laing started to experiment with psychedelics, which Rycroft was strongly opposed to. He was a puritan, and just like many Buddhists, he was of the opinion that working with such substances was like spiritual robbery, where one breaks into a place without having earned a ticket to enter. Although in the history of humanity, various psychotropic substances have always accompanied spirituality and religious experiences, they were always used within the framework of a living culture, as part of the community, of the ritual. However, we do not have a culture like that, we only have egoistic individual initiatives, and we don't possess the necessary tradition. This was important for Rycroft. In South America, the whole village gathers for the ritual of the ayahuasca shaman, the whole community participates in it. We only have quasi-communities, like people waiting for a train or bus, standing in a queue, travelling and then separating. These extemporary communities don't stay together. There is no continuation. Rycroft believed that because of these differences, we shouldn't attempt those same drugs. But Laing was strong in his views that, either you cannot do anything, since every prohibition is incidental, the result of consensual morality or the momentary conviction of an individual, or you can do everything. Whatever is not forbidden is allowed. Everything is allowed, everything is permitted up to the point we agree on among ourselves. I think he regretted the breakup because they didn't speak again. Most people are not aware of how influential Rycroft was as a thinker. Laing once told me that looking back at his life, he didn't have many regrets, but he did lament spending several years in analysis because the whole thing was a brainwashing exercise. He had to work so hard to climb out of the matrix he had been crammed into. Both Winnicott and Rycroft worked in a system, they worked within dogmas. During his years of analysis with both of them, Laing acquired thought conventions and patterns. It took a lot of hard work to challenge and break out of them. Still, I had to tediously work my way through everything. He deemed that important when he was teaching me.

My philosophical family starts with Socrates (not Aristotle!), then moves to Blaise Pascal, Michel de Montaigne (not Descartes!), Søren Kierkegaard, Wittgenstein and Sartre. Laing worked and reflected a lot with David Cooper[1], and it was a very brotherly, horizontal relationship between them. They studied and translated Sartre into English together. Cooper was a very radical thinker too, and his books also became important to me. Later, Cooper moved to France and he and Laing parted ways. Cooper crossed boundaries in his practice Laing would never have crossed. Laing never took advantage of his patients in any way. He considered any form of exploitation unacceptable. But Cooper slept with his patients, moved in with the family, and slept with everyone, one by one, or all over the place, both men and women. Laing eventually told him to fuck off. He wanted to have nothing more to do with him. The Skeptics are also a significant branch of this family for me. They were the therapists of the classical Greeks, and they believed that dogmatists suffered because they were attached to their convictions.[2] This connects to Laing's favourite question, mentioned previously, which he often asked me or himself: "Are you sure about that?" He was the only teacher of mine who asked "what shall we do when we don't know what to do?" John Heaton wrote about this branch of the family in his book, *The Talking Cure*.[3]

Among phenomenologists, Edmund Husserl and Maurice Merleau-Ponty are not easy to read, but their books, *Logical Investigations* by Husserl and *Sense and Non-Sense* by Merleau-Ponty, are worth working through. *Guru*, by Sheldon Kopp, is also important because it describes the anthropology of psychotherapy, the role of priests, rabbis and healers. It gave me a perspective that I could explore deeply with Francis Huxley. I saw Huxley practically as much as I saw Laing in London, and I took my dreams to him. Huxley used to walk up and down in his huge library, and depending on my dream, he recommended books to read. Thus, my anthropological studies were guided by Huxley's interpretations of my dreams. In June 2016, I visited him in San Francisco. We were happy to see each other. He was 92, and we had known each other for 44 years. He was a fragile old man, he moved slowly with the help of a cane and he was hard of hearing, yet he was witty, eloquent and polite. He made me a cup of tea, we had a little wine, and I fetched some sushi from a nearby restaurant. We laughed and reminisced a lot, and we said a very tender goodbye. After all, who knew if we would ever see each other again.[4]

JOURNAL ENTRIES,

1974–75, London

I arrive in London on September first, 1974.

I get to know Hugh Crawford first. He is a Scottish psychiatrist and a good friend of Ronnie's. He is a member of the Philadelphia Association. I approach him with my questions. I muster the courage to ask them, and he replies that he doesn't know who he is talking to. I am standing there, 34 years old, and I have no idea what just happened. How should I tell him who I am? "Not every question has an answer. There are questions that are impossible to answer," he says, "especially if I don't know who I am talking to." Well, this isn't a great start. Or is it?

During the last 42 years or more, on several occasions, I started therapy with a new patient in a similar way: I sit quietly, I turn towards them, I am open, accepting, and I listen. If the silence goes on very long, and I can sense the patient feeling anxious, I gently tell them that I don't know them yet, and so I can't really ask them anything personal. But they approached me, so something must be hurting. They must be suffering from something. Maybe they can introduce themselves by explaining what prompted them to see me.

I meet John Heaton next, who unexpectedly asks me if I have read Merleau-Ponty and how much Freud I have read. With his questions, he is trying to figure out whether I am a behaviourist, and whether I know what transference is. "A therapist will either work with transference, or they are a behaviourist," he says. He wants to know my goal, and I am naive enough to tell him that I want to discover new things. He sneers. "There is nothing new under the sun," he says. "You just don't have enough knowledge and experience." That is, for him, the only explanation for me thinking there are any new things to discover. The whole discussion is awfully demoralising.

Fortunately, I soon get to know Francis Huxley. He tells me to ignore Heaton. "Yes, yes, everything is one, everything is connected to everything else, nothing happens by chance and nothing is original," he says, but tells me I can still be original. "Humanity has known the truths since time immemorial, but these truths have to be articulated anew. Each generation needs a different manner of articulation, and the truths can be expressed through art, science or psychology." Huxley encourages and inspires me. He recommends some books to read, including anything by Géza Róheim and W.B. Yeats' autobiography. Yeats used hypnosis in his poetry. Huxley knows that I am interested in hypnosis, and Yeats used to hypnotise his wife. He wrote down what she said in hypnosis and published her words under his own name.

I meet Leon Redler. He suggests I start practising zazen and Aikido, and that I should play music and sing.

Later on, Laing often played the piano, and I was invited to sing Hungarian folk songs. I sat many zazens with Leon Redler but

Aikido never agreed with me. I don't like it when my body is black and blue and everything hurts.

Momentous day. I meet Laing, and he introduces me to the casual, dogma-free Philadelphia Association, and the five people who manage the houses: Laing, Crawford, Heaton, Huxley and Redler. Their relationship is not formalised; there is no bureaucracy.

Laing asserts that he is not against medication. Lithium can be beneficial in many cases. He is not an irresponsible doctor who will leave a diabetic without their insulin. If a psychiatrist recommends some medicine to him, he is happy to try it himself. He always reminds his patients that the responsibility belongs to them. They should be attentive to see if they are well, and the doctor should pay attention to what their patient says. The doctor is just a counsellor; the patient should have the power. If a patient wants medication, then Laing will find another doctor who is familiar with medicines and sends the person to them. His relationship with his patients is not medical.

I have the same position in relation to EMDR (the technique of eye movement desensitisation and reprocessing is used for treating traumas). I find applying it very boring, but if that's what the person wants, I send them to Marshall Wilensky, a professional practitioner. I don't want to do it because me being the knower, the expert, changes the transference, the relationship. Marshall likes to be an expert, and he makes use of this proclivity. For him, the important thing is being the expert, not the sense of a relationship. That's not a problem, but in therapy, there is no knowledge and no experts. If I act like an expert on anything, then transference will last much longer because the patients are socialised to be led by someone. Therapy is about accompanying someone, not leading them. There are many experts working at the Feldmár Institute: counsellors, trainers, coaches, superb experts and professionals. This is acceptable because we also have carpenters, but what they do is not therapy. A person teaching and nurturing is not talking with someone, just as a person employing a technique is not talking with someone. Real conversation isn't didactic. It doesn't have a predetermined goal, and it doesn't want to convince anyone of anything. We come together in language, we allow language to speak us, and we open up to each other with curiosity and affection, careful not to lose each other, careful to keep our relationship alive. I was always suspicious of Socrates. He wanted to guide others to where he already knew what the truth was. Therapy is not like that. I have hope that genuine things are put into words, emerge between us, and then we can both be surprised.

I visit one of the shelters. A man is dozing in a sleeping bag. We start chatting. He is angry. He says, "The shelter is no good, it's shit. Laing is like an Edwardian lord, a tyrant with 18–20 kids. Paul Zeal and Haya Oakley are like step-parents. They weaken the community. Zeal is the dick, Oakley is the tits, and as an authentic revolutionary action, Oakley and Zeal should both be fucked, raped. And therapy is just masturbation or sex in disguise." I am thrown off balance, but I let him be. I tell him, "That's OK," and I don't argue with him. This is my first time in such a house. I am shocked. It's exciting, frightening, and rough, all at the same time.

I have so much to do. I am reading Claudio Naranjo's *The One Quest* and Roberto Assagioli's *The Act of Will*. I read about snot in *Voices* magazine[1], and I start practising yoga. Yoga is very painful. Through the pain, I become aware of my boundaries and how limited I am. I hate pain, so the chances of change are minimal. I want to change without pain. Mina, my yoga teacher, hurts me gently. Mina has been in therapy with Ronnie for four years. Ronnie had been in analysis with D.W. Winnicott for five years. Mina says Ronnie is her perfect mirror. He always reflects things without distorting them. I go to Ronnie and tell him yoga makes me hurt all over. "The body is for colliding with everything. You don't need to take care of the body," he says. "If one takes care of oneself a great deal, that's a projection that possibly started within the womb, when one is scared of what one may bump into. Thus, one can avoid all exciting collisions."

A boundary may be experienced softly and gently, yet firmly, or every collision may be as painful as a sudden bolt of lightning, almost fatal and excruciating. "Only those who will risk going too far can possibly find out how far one can go."[2] If the first encounter with the lining of the mother's womb is unpleasant, painful or creates a sense of rejection, the organism starts to be frightened of collisions.

"Whether you believe it or not," Ronnie says, "there are people who feel at home in the world." He is obviously talking about me not feeling at home in the world. "Fuck off." We talk about

89

experiences when we are one and experiences when we are separated. Which one is an illusion, which one is real? In his skeptical tradition, there is no answer, but the question is great. There are things that exist simultaneously, not "either/or" but "and". Wilfred Bion[3] says that, in a group, in a community, each member projects their own mother on the group, and those who feel excluded were shunned by their mother. Their mother didn't provide a sense of togetherness. If the mother frustrates the baby too soon, when they grow up, they will be terribly frightened of separateness because the baby has this sense of not being able to exist as an entity separate from their mother. But if the mother is very attentive to how far the baby can be frustrated, then everything is fine. Then, the baby understands that there is the other, and there is oneself. I draw up a map, with Ronnie, about the location of pain, the memory of pain, the memory of hurt, and liberation from hurt. Those for whom it takes a long time to remember how brutal their father or mother were, have to first remember the pain. The memory of pain hurts almost as badly as the pain itself. This was the direction Buddha took, and enlightenment is actually becoming free from the memories of pain.

It is difficult for me here because I often feel ignorant, lazy and stupid. For example, when I talk with an analyst from Mexico who studied in Erich Fromm's school, I feel uneducated and uninformed.

I visit another shelter and meet another therapist, Robin Cooper, who doesn't want me to join the yoga practice held by Mina three times a week for those living at the shelter. After the exercises, everyone relaxes, and that's the reason Robin is reluctant to allow me to join in. He is afraid or fears for the others that I, being a stranger, will make it harder for the others to relax. Mina fortunately convinces him, so I can come here to practise.

I am terribly, insanely curious. Those I meet from Laing's circle, it seems to me, are full of energy and joie de vivre. I am really attracted to this whole thing. I'd like to be one of them. I'd like to belong to them. For the first time in my life, I meet people I value and respect. It's like finding my homeland. Almost everyone seems likeable, and somehow, I have faith that even if something is hard and painful, they will tell me honestly. They are not just out to torture me. I am especially intrigued by the houses, the shelters, despite the fact that it is terrifying that lunatics live there with no one to control them. I am scared, but I want to learn to not be scared, and slowly, I manage to do just that. There are lots of brilliant discussions. There are always a few people sitting around one kitchen table or another, and people are always having tea somewhere and talking. Apart from Robin Cooper, everyone welcomes me. I get to know the third house, where Mary Barnes used to live. Joe Berke, her therapist, later wrote a book with Mary about her journey. Mary went into regression in one of the rooms here, and she made paintings with her own faeces. She doesn't go into regression any more, and she showed me her real paintings that weren't done with shit. She tells me about all of them in an analytical and ultra-critical fashion. She explains what is what. She is a friendly and gentle woman. She has no interest in me, but she is pleased that I am paying attention to her. She wears a long red skirt, her long hair is loose, and she has broad hips. I get the impression of talking with a precocious ten-year-old.

I practise yoga, and my nose gets close to the carpet. I smell shit. Mary Barnes painted her shit-pictures in this room. Ronnie comes, and just like any other time he visits a house, he immediately sits down to play the piano. He starts playing, the others get the instruments out, sing, and the music begins. "Don't complain, don't explain, don't apologise, and don't admit to anything!" Ronnie tells me. I am sure this can only apply to certain situations and not others. The quote is originally from Benjamin Disraeli: "Never complain and never explain."[4] Ronnie adds the other two directives for situations when the other person demands you to do so. What Disraeli meant is that only children have the right to complain, and the need to explain, because they are powerless. These are not laws, but Ronnie constantly thinks about them, conjecturing because they are connected to power or powerlessness somehow. I tell him that when my wife complains, I feel I have a job to do, and he tells me that's because I am stupid. "You have to listen to her like you listen to Wagner. Just hear the music, don't try to solve it," he says. That's it. I feel immediately relieved. My wife's troubles don't bother me so much! He also tells me not to explain anything, as the "why did you do it?" question is completely idiotic. Children, and even adults, never, or hardly ever, know why they do things, but if they are forced, they'll make up a reason. Each explanation is a fiction.

I practise yoga with Mina. She talks a lot. "One shouldn't just practise the poses," she says, "one has to learn to be healthy without feeling guilty about it. So, if I look after myself and others, I deserve to travel the world, to eat, drink and move healthily without feeling guilty." She quotes Patanjali about Buddha speaking to an assembly of people who were healthy. They could sit without pain or fidgeting.

Leon and Haya try to scare me into going back to Canada. "You won't be able to make money here, so you should come back when you have made money in Canada," they say. They also say it would be better not to have Ronnie as my therapist because he travels a lot. He is hardly ever here, and in six months, he will say, "You want to be a therapist? Maybe after seven years of analysis, it may be plausible." I think it's not easy for either of them to keep their head above water in London. It's not easy to make enough money to live here. Maybe they feel their business is threatened, like I am a rival. But I listen to no one and carry on.

Ronnie tells me, during these first few weeks I am in London, that the expression on my face is like someone who has to carry heavy weights. Weights I don't even want, but I am not assertive enough, so I keep apologising for being me. I have an apologetic face, he tells me, as if I am not valuable enough to deserve another's attention. My voice is gentle. Maybe I hide my aggression behind gentleness. He thinks I can just change my voice and gait. I move here and there, left and right, not straightforwardly, not directly ahead.

It's important for a therapist to teach the patient how to tell others to leave them alone, or more precisely, how to say, "Let me be!" or "Get off my back!" It is only possible if the therapist models this behaviour with solid, hard boundaries: this far, and no further. It is stating "now you are in my private sphere, whether it is a visual sphere, audio, tactile or olfactory sphere. I am the lord and master of distance in my space. I tell you how close you can approach me in these spheres." The lemma is not allowing the patient, even for a moment, to break into any of my spheres.[5] It's not good for him, and it's not good for me.

Leon reads me excerpts from his journal, from 1966 to '68. He reads me his letters, dreams and notes about his therapy with Ronnie. I am shocked by his honest thoughts. Leon is raging a lot and breaking chairs. I go to Ronnie for therapy and ask him what is wrong with me because I am not raging. He laughs. "There is only one reason," he says, "you are not Leon. You don't do it like Leon." But that doesn't mean anything when I'm looking for direction; there is no schema and no blueprint. It's all new to me.

I relate to a lot of Leon's feelings. We both compare ourselves to Ronnie. We both feel intellectually and creatively dwarfed by Ronnie's giant. We are both struggling with the ambivalence of the unpleasantness and frightening nature of being alone, yet we yearn for aloneness. Both of us are rarely joyful and rarely happy. We can't enjoy the moment. We suffer. I examine and watch myself very rigorously, and in this clever way, I avoid changes. I hide everything from myself. I even hide the fact that I hide things. Leon tries out what it's like to struggle a lot with murderous and suicidal thoughts. We talk about envying our patients sometimes, but then we both just pay attention to what is. We sit and breathe. We become brothers in Ronnie's family.

After zazen one day, I make my way home on the underground, and I fantasise that everyone is watching me and noticing the book I am reading. Then, I realise this fantasy is only about women, as if each woman is my mother. I am urging her to take notice of me, to love me, to pay attention to me. I do everything for my mother. It goes like this: "I can't be alone because I always want more of you! Look how smart I am. If you don't pay attention, I won't do anything… Oh no!"

Laing shows me a Diane Arbus photo of a young boy holding a hand grenade. His body is all tensed up. Ronnie says he reminded him of me. There is some aggressive and destructive energy about the picture, but it is tamed and suppressed.

I have a cold, but I still go for Mina's yoga practice. She has been in therapy with Ronnie for four years, and she is now weaning herself off. Sometimes, she goes back for a cuddle. I read Carlos Castaneda and Claudio Naranjo. Stanley Keleman[6] speaks about the two ways of dying: opening the doors wide, even reaching out to death; or being attached to life and holding onto the smallest spark of life until the last possible moment. I think I belong to the first category. As you live, so you die. Thrifty people die slowly. My father, for example, first lost his hearing, then his vision, then he had to be put in diapers. He lost one thing after another, and at the end, he was like a small baby. Then he died. I'd rather explode in a heart attack. I'd rather live till the last moment, socially and psychologically undamaged to the very end.

I really like how Ronnie is so courteous and cordial as he works; he is an attentive, caring and polite host. He helps the previous patient with their coat, and he welcomes me in. We arrange that, if one of his patients doesn't mind, I can come, and at the end of the session, Ronnie will hand him or her over to me. I end up with a psychiatrist. He's been working for the navy for five years. He has problems with himself and his wife. His wife attends Leon's therapy, and he usually goes to Hugh Crawford, but he comes to Ronnie for consultation. He is telling us about his dream: he stole something, he was drunk, the police were chasing him, they caught him, he was struggling, but they held him down. To me, it seems that despite degrading himself, he is somehow boasting. His mind goes round in circles, and he can't blurt out why he came to see Ronnie. He is scared of everything he has to let go of. Ronnie asks him what would happen if he let go of everything, and he just fantasises. The guy talks about how reading Ronnie's books saved his life. He cannot be authentic in his work as a doctor. He experiences huge tension: his duties on one side, family and work, and his yearning for freedom on the other side. He never has enough money. He looks away and doesn't look either of us in the eye. He is just squeezing the words out. He is strained and tense. I think about how stealing in a dream could mean one is defrauding oneself. Being drunk is an extenuating circumstance, but he can't get rid of his own guilty conscience, the police. I am more of an observer, so I rarely cut in. I watch Ronnie, and how he relates to his patient. He doesn't try to connect all the dots. He doesn't finish things, and everything remains open. Later on, he explains that nothing needs to be resolved; one has to partake of an experience, authentically. This is the job of the therapist. No need to help, just take part, live in what's there, and give yourself to the situation. All three of us gain experiences. I pay more attention to the atmosphere and less to the details. I observe Ronnie's boundless warmth, openness, and affection. I am a little scared, and a bit anxious. What am I doing here between two psychiatrists? Sometimes I feel like a child among two adults. It really disturbs me at first, then I manage to overcome my fear. I want to be brave. I have a good quality of throwing myself into things, no matter how terrified I might be. I don't want to miss out on any opportunity that comes my way here. Ronnie says I am cultivating, practising, courage. William Blake[7] says that if you are proud of yourself for being able to control your emotions, it may be because what you feel is tiny while others are struggling with enormous, gigantic emotions. Nobody knows the size of others' feelings because it is absolutely subjective and inexorably private.

> I think Blake is possibly right. The ramification is that if I could actually be in someone else's skin, if I could actually become them, then I would do the same things as them. This is the source of a question I often ask myself when one of my patients acts in a bizarre manner: "What circumstances, beliefs, and emotions would prompt me to behave like them?" Since we cannot know people's inner struggles, when we see A being able to control their emotions, while B being unable to do so, we shouldn't hasten to praise A and censure B. A may only have a light breeze of an emotion while in B there is a raging hurricane. Don't compare yourself to others. Everyone has to deal with their own emotions. One may be a dwarf, another a giant. How can you compare the two? My mother often rebuked me, "Why are you not like Árpi?" Because I am Andrew, that's why.

Laing entrusts the guy, the psychiatrist, to me, at the end of the session. I never see him again.

We are all at a seminar by Hugh Crawford, called "I Find Myself in the World." How can I find myself at home? How can I make the world my home? "Style is the key," says Crawford. "My style determines how I exist in the world. It's not that someone from the outside shoved or conjured me into this world. It wasn't a magic feat that brought me into this world from the void. It was one of my mother's cells that started growing. This world grew me from itself. My consciousness was moulded by my mother's consciousness. Physicists consider consciousness to be a state of matter. Matter includes mother: material, *mater*. Matter has solid, liquid and gaseous states, so it can also have a state of consciousness. Or, in other words, consciousness is a state of matter. My mother is such a state of matter, and the guru is like a mother to the student, like a state of consciousness that moulds the consciousness of the disciple." Crawford says, "The guru is a 'mother-rectifier'. Let's start with: I am what the other means to me. I am what my mother means to me or what the guru means."

Generally, there are two ways to think or feel about myself: 1) I am what others mean to me, or 2) I am what I mean to others. The first one is subjective: if I allow others to be important to me, then I am filled with my love, appreciation and joy. The second one is fantasy: I can never understand what I mean to others and to toil for others' love and appreciation is an unending endeavour, a stubbornness and wilfulness, that creates anxiety.

Crawford continues: "The alternative is that I am what I mean to the other. If I am their everything, then I am the universe.

They live in me like we used to live in our mother. So, there is this realisation that through the guru, we get to our mother and through our mother, to God. Guru, mother, me: this is how we grasp that we are one. I find myself when the other person is my everything. This is where love and attention come from, and whatever I notice, happens in this spirit." Mina takes the floor and tells us that the first time she felt loved was when she got to know Ronnie, at the age of 35. Ronnie was happy for her every little success and tolerated her old weaknesses. She felt like Ronnie had been her mother, a mother who was totally accepting; a good mother.

The seminar room is too crowded, too hot, and I can hardly breathe. Crawford speaks slowly and hesitantly, with lots of pauses. The whole thing is freaking awkward and uncomfortable. It's not a good place, yet it's exciting and stimulating. Mina says she didn't feel at home because, up to that point, she hadn't been sure if she could interrupt to say something. For a child who feels at home, it's not even a question. Somewhere, she lost this child-like "at home" feeling. Crawford makes a distinction between self-discipline and obligation. He says "the less we sense the relationship and ties with each other, the more we live by rules. The worse the relationship, the more rules you need. If it's a good community with strong relationships, then we look out for each other, care for each other, everything regulates itself and we feel free." Then he sends us home to read Maurice Merleau-Ponty. I read Epictetus, Spinoza and Nietzsche.

David Goldblatt, the American, is here with his family, like I am with mine. We are Ronnie's twins. David is familiar with the situation. He's been here for a while, and he introduces me to

London and London to me. We are alike, and we become close. We talk about Christ, psychoanalysis, and the first letter of the Kabbalah, *aleph*. David believes our birth continues at every moment. We are constantly being born and of course constantly dying, as well. We talk about marriage, sex, and why we shouldn't have sex with patients. This, of course, should be obvious, but we feel attractions here and there. I always get the sense of stifled sobs in the sound of his voice. He sees me as a timid person. He thinks he, Mina, I and Ronnie are one in the sense that we are looking for something else, something more; we are not satisfied with what is.

I take some of my dreams about mirror reflections to Ronnie. He shows me some poems he wrote about mirrors and takes out a manuscript he will soon publish. He tells me that once he was a rat in a dream. He was dying of the plague in a Hong Kong sewer. He believes that the mirror motif takes us back to conception. First, we are one cell, and when we divide into two, it is like mirroring each other. This goes on until we become a small set of cells, a ball. This terrible, constant division is present in our life until we bury it, until we dig in, until we become embedded in our mother's womb. That's where we finally lose our symmetry. "Each relationship starts," he says, "like conception. Its duration is the pregnancy, and there is birth at the end." It is particularly great to apply this notion to therapy: the patient is conceived when they step through the door, therapy is the pregnancy and the end of therapy is birth.

Ronnie suggests that the style of a relationship may be related to our experiences in the womb. If at the beginning of pregnancy, the mother is unsure about keeping her foetus, it is possible that the person experiences or repeats this uncertainty at the beginning of each new relationship. The beginning may be full of anxiety, then the relationship warms up and ecstasy comes as the mother accepts her embryo and enjoys the happiness of expectancy. Or, it is not unusual that the person conceives of or formulates an idea, wants to do something, the idea is growing, the person envisions how they could accomplish it, works out all the details in their mind, but never brings it into the world, never gives birth to anything. There are some thoughts that fail to embed. The thought comes, it grows, then it is lost. Maybe embedding was difficult.

"It is not actually sex that I want from a woman. I want to see myself in her. I am looking for a mirror reflection." Hugh Crawford is talking. I am at his seminar. "Trauma stops or checks growing up or development. It arrests growth. When something terrible happens in the womb, the organism stalls or becomes stuck in a particular state and doesn't register later events," he says. He tells us about a 30-year-old man who, as if he had never been born, lost all the experiences that happened from birth to the age of three because they were recorded somewhere else.

When a promise is broken, it is very difficult to remedy. The damage created by a broken promise may be permanent. Lies generate bad karma because we deny reality from the other person, but they still perceive reality, through their pores, through their body, because every vibration contains the truth. Jealousy is fine, and open marriages are also fine, if the partners can tolerate the thought of their spouse's genitals coming in contact with another person's. Hugh has encountered many people for whom this is unbearable.

The word "speculate" comes from *speculum,* which means "mirror" in Latin.[8] Astronomers used to study heavenly bodies with various mirrors. They used to examine and speculate. Hugh tells us he once saw a man at a bar twisting his leg behind his neck after dinner, giving himself a blowjob. He spoke about Ronnie, too, and said he lives in cycles, and he keeps getting into a phase where there is too much wine, whisky, hash, self-gratification and self-indulgence.

I attend Francis Huxley's seminar, and he speaks about honesty, integrity and dignity. Francis is tall, and he has an impressive face with sharp features, resembling Aldous Huxley, his uncle. Just like me, Huxley only uses one eye, and if I look at his sightless eye, I get an odd feeling; I don't know where he is looking. If I switch to his seeing eye, he is watching, seeing, connected. He says there are lots of one-eyed shamans in Brazil. He speaks with a deep voice, doesn't pronounce his r's, and is exceptionally eloquent. He gesticulates and laughs a lot. His sense of humour is similar to Ronnie's, bordering on the cynical.

When one cannot achieve the ideal ego or ego-ideal, which comes from our parents, society and peers of course, one feels ashamed. Listening to Francis, I realise that when I measure myself against this ideal me and I turn out to be less, I feel shame. Guilt, on the other hand, is something else. When I break something or disobey the orders of the superego, I feel guilty. Of course, the superego also comes from our parents and predecessors, says Francis. Shame, therefore, is related to the ego-ideal while guilt is connected to the superego. The superego tells us what's allowed and what's forbidden. Disobeying it is a matter of morality. Ego-ideal relates to my being, what kind of person I am. These two, guilt and shame, feel different and appear in different places in the body. According to Francis, the word "shame" is etymologically related to the French word *chemise*, "shirt". A shirt is for covering nakedness, what we feel ashamed of. In other words, fashion is an opportunity to be proud of the things we cover our shame with. The more you try to adorn what you are trying to hide away, the more you feel ashamed of what you want to conceal. The essence, the most crucial point, is that shame is related to my being while guilt is connected to my actions.

"Shame on you!" is much worse, deeper and more permanent than "Alas, what have you done?!" Shame designates you: that's what you are, you can't do anything about it. Guilt or remorse ends when I stop doing the wrong things and try to rectify my mistakes. I am a thief: this is destiny, fate that I inherited, there is no way out. I stole: well, I could stop doing that.

Etymologically, "guilt" includes the Latin *torquere*, which means "to twist". The root word is *tort*, injury, damage, being wronged. So, it is connected to vice, evil, guilt and turd, which also happens to twist.[9] The large intestine also twists, going from right to left before ending in the rectum. According to Francis, this bodily structure creates the association that gives a bad connotation to "left." This is an example showing that we must deal with language, words and meanings constantly because we live in the language. We dream and associate in the language. Honour can create conceit, and shame may originate from yearning to become great but failing. Excommunication, ostracism, is the greatest shame. Falling out of others' hearts, goodwill, everybody turning away from one, is also shame. Thus, shame is related to good and bad, whereas guilt is connected to things done well and badly. When a child is doing something, it's a *performance*, and if they are told to stop that immediately, it creates shame. The child is having a pee or a poo, or even laughing, and is told to stop. Someone snaps at them: "What do you think you are doing?!" or "You're not doing it properly!" The child feels shame and embarrassment. They feel self-conscious and start looking at themself as if someone else is doing the looking. Interruption per se is shame-inducing.

According to Spinoza, shame is the pain one experiences for being the cause of something bad. In the case of pride, joy is associated with being the cause. If being the cause is painful, then it is shame, and if being the cause is pleasing, then that is pride. Francis agrees and tells us that in certain cultures, tribes and peoples, one is allowed to work off shame and guilt, and in others, once you are disgraced, there is no way out; the culture doesn't let you escape the shame.

Francis offers us an example. Southeast Asia celebrates the Thaipusam festival, where one million people go for atonement every year, around the end of January. The festival commemorates the goddess Parvati giving a spear to her son, who killed an evil demon with it. It is a great celebration that originates from the story of a saint, Idumban, carrying two mountains on his shoulders when he met the son of Svaha who acted impudently.

Idumban was enraged and the two mountains suddenly became so heavy that he could hardly carry them. When he realised who the insolent boy was (Kartikeya) and atoned, his burden became light again. During the festival, people carry heavy burdens like large goblets full of milk, and they are not allowed to spill even a drop. They walk 15 kilometres to the temple, climb a hill that is full of caves, and fall into a trance. They pierce their tongue and cheeks with small spears, and they stick hooks in their backs to pull heavy weights up the 272 steps to the altar that they sprinkle with milk. And they feel good afterwards.

"So," says Francis, "there are cultures that allow for atonement, remorse, but we don't have that any more. Public confessions are replaced by a confession box, but that doesn't really alleviate the shame because confessions become impersonal. One can be a spiritual person, but one cannot fail to include the psyche. One has to confess one's sins to God, but in the company of others. There is a mechanism: if you do such and such, you accumulate more sins, but next year, you can become free from them. We prefer to get sick." He continues, "One of my patients is very hard on himself. He is very strict with himself. He is dissatisfied: he should be very successful, but he is not, and he hates himself. He and his wife went for a European tour. The day they arrived in Paris, he fainted, his throat constricted and he almost died. To this day, he has a terrible cough and can hardly talk. He was punishing himself because he didn't deserve to enjoy Europe, because he wasn't as famous and successful as he should have been. He compares himself to someone else, and if he is less than the paragon, he will kill himself like Hemingway, who was also dissatisfied with himself for not being masculine enough and stuck a gun in his mouth. My answer to this patient is it is better to kill his ideals, but to him that would be a kind of shameful escapism, and I don't know what would have to happen for him to love himself as he is. This is self-punishment. He is strict and harsh with himself to the extreme. It is a narcissistic wound that he can't achieve everything by his willpower. He is wounded, and he can't and doesn't want to survive this."

Haya Oakley's seminar is about one of Winnicott's papers, "Hate in the Counter-Transference".[10] He wrote it in 1947. It's a crucial piece of work. Winnicott writes about how children and lunatics don't believe that someone loves them if that person can't hate them when the child or lunatic mistreats them. According to him, if you don't express when something hurts, when someone upsets you, if you can't be angry, if you constantly smile, then they won't believe you when things are genuinely fine. Children and lunatics turn away from a person who is unable to sometimes be angry, who is unable to occasionally hate, because they don't believe that the person is able to love. So, the therapist must be genuine. When the patient hurts them, they have to express precisely how they feel. Winnicott worked with babies, children and lunatics. He was a doctor, a pediatrician, as well as a psychoanalyst. His observations come from great depths. The significant difference between psychoanalysis and existential analysis is that, in psychoanalysis, the therapist uses transference to deny the reality of the patient's emotions, and so it results in frustration. According to Freud, therapists shouldn't have emotions. According to an existential therapist like Medard Boss,[11] the patient's emotions are always real. Existential phenomenology doesn't forbid you from feeling, thinking or believing in particular things; it tries to accurately describe what is.

I am not looking for an explanation, but I am trying to understand the other person, empathise with their world, just like when I read a poem. I allow it to carry me wherever it is pointing to. The patient and the poet both try to say something that words are not adequate to express. We have to look in the direction they are pointing in. You can't practise analysis with psychotic or schizophrenic patients if you, the analyst, don't take your own emotions seriously, even the momentary awakening of hatred towards the patient. The therapist has to vocalise what they are going through, how they feel in the company of their patient, otherwise they will explode with rage, aggression, helplessness and/or frustration. This explains why they used to treat patients with incredible brutality in old lunatic asylums. They hated them, but it wasn't even a subject of discussion. They didn't even recognise that they were punishing patients because they didn't understand them. According to Winnicott, one who can't accept their own hatred shouldn't work with lunatics. A lunatic's love and hatred can both be terribly dangerous and frightening. They simultaneously love and hate their therapist. For recovery, it is important that the patient has had at least a few pleasant experiences in the past. If they go through their first good experiences with the therapist, then every small detail is significant, everything is scrutinised under a microscope. They pay close attention because they can't believe that the therapist is different from those who hurt them in the past. They look and hunt for a mistake the therapist may make. If they think the therapist is only nice with them for the money, the relationship, the therapy doesn't work. But if the therapist can become angry when the situation calls for it, the patient will have confidence in the good experiences. Even they wouldn't think that someone would lose their temper for money.

According to Haya, in reality a mother will feel hatred towards her baby before the baby could hate their mother. A mother often feels that she is forced to love the baby, as if someone held a gun to her head, forcing her. There is a child in her fantasy and a child in reality, and the two children are different. When she was dreaming about having a child, she wasn't yearning for the child that appeared. But a good mother and a good therapist must be able to tolerate their negative emotions, and they have to liberate themselves to be able to accept these without guilt. This doesn't mean that they can pour their unbridled anger on the child or patient, but that they tolerate it in themselves, and they don't hide it from their child or patient. But if this is never communicated, the child or patient will have to feel indebted to the mother or therapist. A good therapist doesn't just heal but wounds too, or at least they indicate that they feel like wounding now, in this situation.

I am about to finish the book *Hara*, by Karlfried Graf Dürckheim. He speaks about the vital centre of the human, located five centimetres under the navel, and he calls it *tanden*. Stubbornness, wilfulness, causes suffering. A human's duty is to become what they are. A master has achieved this unity one hundred percent, not just occasionally, but permanently. Dürckheim uses the metaphor of an archer: one has mastered archery if they can always hit the bullseye, not just occasionally but every single time. If they shoot several arrows and they hit and split their previous arrow, they, the target, the bow and the arrow are all one. They can use their bow like I can touch my nose with my finger. Beyond everything that is important for my ego, there is a deeper spiritual desire related to my entirety, not just my ego. So, the ego shouldn't be eradicated because, if we pay attention, we can find morsels of the great truth in the ego. Dürckheim says that in every spiritual practice: the first lesson already contains everything, but a beginner is unable to experience it. Their curiosity will lead them to ask what is the most, the highest one can achieve by this practice.

I have a conversation with Ronnie. He shows me *Laws of Form* by G. Spencer-Brown. The guy is a mathematician who taught Ronnie algebra and mathematics in return for Ronnie's therapy sessions. John C. Lilly[12] spent weeks on the first page of this book. This is the kind of book it is. Ronnie wanted to open this math door that was closed for him in school because if the parents or teachers declare it, a child will believe that they are not talented in this or that subject. This is all psycho-hypnotic suggestion, but it can be called a curse just as easily. The only way to come out of it is with a person who is really good at that subject, lifting the curse. Ronnie removed my curse of not being able to sing because of being called "tone-deaf." When the curse is broken, inhibition ceases and presto, one immediately enjoys doing that particular thing. I am telling Ronnie how the number three appeared in my dream, and we talk about the significance of three in my life. I was three when my mother left me, there were three people in my family: three with my father, mother and me; I had three wives; my father also had three wives. Three crops up a lot in my dreams. Then he says I am responsible for my face. I think Jean-Paul Sartre has already said that. Laing thinks the more I accept my body, the more I am unconcerned by it, the more hair I'll allow to grow. First my face was bare, then I had a moustache, then a beard and a moustache, then a beard, moustache and shaggy hair. He also sometimes has a moustache, beard, or both.

David Goldblatt tells me that he met up with Ronnie just before my session. He wanted to tell him how much he loved and respected him, but the words wouldn't come out. For the entire hour, David sat cross-legged and cried. He was looking at Ronnie, who didn't look at him and didn't say anything. He hardly ever said anything to him. Once, Ronnie even fell asleep in the middle of the session. He woke up because of some ringing from the street. They never discussed this. David didn't bring it up, and Ronnie didn't apologise. Once, Ronnie didn't accept money for one of the sessions. When David arrived, Ronnie showed him a newspaper article about a guy who was playing the guitar and was executed in front of his fans. First, they broke all his fingers, then they killed him. Ronnie was weeping while he read the article and then just sat down to play the piano, and they sang together. He didn't accept money for this. David and I agree that Ronnie never does anything for theoretical reasons, he just is, he just exists, lives.

I start my own practice in London. My first patient arrives. He is a moustachioed young man, wearing trainers. He is Steve, 27 years old. His parents divorced when he was very little and he was brought up by his father, a Hungarian chap, and his Catholic grandmother. How did he end up with me? Curious. He had a seven-year relationship with a woman who was four years older than him. He is single now and very uncertain. The woman switched to a lesbian relationship. That was the reason for leaving him, and Steve blames the feminist movement for this. He feels emasculated, as if he lost his manhood. He is not homosexual, but he is in a homoerotic relationship with a friend. Recently, he was high on some drugs and got terrified that this friend could rape him. Now, he is not even sure whether he is a boy or a girl. He feels he is running away. He is hiding from men and from women, also. He is studying movie animation at art college, constantly torments himself, and is not sure about anything. He practices yoga and meditation but not regularly, and he is constantly anxious about how others see him. He doesn't look at the world through his own eyes. He had a few affairs, but he kept them secret from his girl. Still, when his partner started publicly dating women, Steve became insanely angry and hurt. I observe him and notice how he is so different from me and so much like me.

I watch Peter Robinson's movie, *Asylum*. It was made in one of the London shelters. One of the scenes touches me deeply: a girl is playing the guitar and keeps singing "wake up, wake up", and she relaxes completely. I start crying. After the film, I go to Mina's for a late dinner and party. There are quite a few people there from the Philadelphia Association. It's as if the movie continued. I get this sense that Ronnie is everywhere, since nearly everyone attends his therapy, and those who don't, still know him, keep note of him, and take their cue from him. We are his patients or students, and we feel that he is amongst us. But now, at this party, there is a writer present, Jakov Lind. He doesn't seem to like Ronnie. There is an infamous story: Jakov had a party and everyone brought some food. Ronnie and his wife Jutta brought a salad in a dish. When the party had finished, and they were about to leave, Jakov told them that there was still some food in the dish, and he would return it the next time he visited them. Jutta impressed on Jakov how important the dish was to her, and how he shouldn't forget about it. When Jakov went to see them a couple of weeks later, Jutta asked him where the dish was. Jakov was rude enough to tell her to give him a break about the dish. He threw his keys at Jutta and told her to go and find it herself if it is so important to her. Ronnie took the keys, flung them back at Jakov and told him "If the dish is not here within an hour, never darken our doorstep ever again." The dish was there within half an hour. But from that time on, Jakov has been really vindictive behind Ronnie's back. I think he is jealous of Ronnie's youthfulness, energy and joie de vivre because they are of the same age, but Jakov seems much older. Ronnie becomes like the person he is with to the extent that he doesn't seem to have his own character. He reflects the other person's character, so everyone has his own Ronnie, different from everyone else's.

Later, in April 2009, a street in Vienna was named after Jakov: Jakov-Lind-Strasse.

I am reading Winnicott's book, *The Child, the Family, and the Outside World,* and one of Francis Huxley's books. Francis wrote it in 1956, when he lived with the Urubu natives in Brazil.[13] Winnicott writes about how parents often don't believe that they are good enough to create a normal, beautiful little baby. Winnicott encourages new parents to get to know their child because the more they pay attention to them, the more positively the baby can teach them that, yes, this perfection came from them.

I go for a therapy session with Ronnie. I feel anxious and uneasy, and I don't know why. Ronnie, as if he senses this, is very comforting, kind, warm and gentle. He reacts to everything by listening very carefully. We talk about the past. His hypothesis is that when my mother was taken when I was three, I closed the door behind her and never let her in again. And I did the same thing with my father and my grandmother as well. When they came back, nothing was ever the same, we couldn't go back to where we were before we were separated. He says the more I relax, the better it gets. The road always leads towards relaxation. I can't forcefully want something. If I relax, I can go down to where the trauma happened, and then I'll be able to let it go, I'll be able to turn off the alarm bells that were switched on inside me. He remembers a few moments when he locked people out because they hurt him. Every compulsive action is an excellent opportunity for good observations. If you examine something, you can find its origin. It occurs to me that I wind my family's watches, all of them – my kids', my wife's, I operate everyone's watches. What could this be? Where does it come from? "Carry on," says Ronnie, "don't stop, but pay attention to what you feel, why it feels good, and you will recognise yourself." I shouldn't have an opinion of myself, I should just be curious about my associations, emotions that emerge when I wind up the watches. Just like recurring dreams stop recurring when you understand their meaning, such compulsive actions also discontinue by themselves once one manages to dig out all possible meanings. Maybe I am that species of tiny animal-humans who enjoys touching everything, I want to hold everyone's watches? That's fine, I don't have to stop, but I should be careful not to expect others' gratitude for doing something because I like it.

> A few months later, I noticed that the kids got angry with me because their watches stopped. That showed me a change had taken place. I told them that from then on it was their job. I gave them back the responsibility.

The thing I have to realise, to decide to know, is that I don't have to do anything no matter what I feel, no matter what impulses may come. In the gap between impulse and doing, or doing nothing, I can find the difference between what the reality was in the past, and what is just a memory or fantasy of it now. It is crucial to pay attention. I say goodbye to someone, and I get angry or feel like crying, but I don't go after them, I don't do anything. At this moment in time, I realise that every goodbye takes me back to the time when my mother, father, and grandmother disappeared for a long time.

> One of my patients, from the Maritimes, used to work as a waiter in a restaurant, but he was caught hiding a camera in the ladies' toilet, filming women peeing and pooping. He came to me for therapy. He couldn't understand why he did this. He

knew it was very foolish, pointless, and dangerous; still, he felt a deep sense of satisfaction for being able to spy on what women did behind closed doors. He was in an orphanage for a long time, then a family adopted him. The mother loved him greatly, and because he was always scared, he could follow her wherever she went, even to the toilet. But at a certain point, the woman told him that he was a big boy now and closed the toilet door in front of him. He couldn't imagine what his mother was doing behind the closed door. And now, there is a 27-year-old man standing before me who fucked up his career, and his partner left him, because he gave himself up to this feeling, this impulse. If he would have paid attention to his feelings, he could have realised what was going on, but he acted out, and created big trouble. The pressure of unresolved, unexpressed, frozen traumas is inevitable. Where we have a choice is whether to act it out or work it through.

With Ronnie again. We talk about my fear that basically, deep down, I am just a piece of shit. A lot of people, maybe everyone, is afraid of this. Ronnie says it may just be confusion because for all intents and purposes, the child could come from the same place as shit, from the intestines, through their mother's arse and not her cunt, and that there is some dreamlike equation between bones, shit, and death. Bones are hidden, and so is shit – everything that's already dead. He says that, for the last three years, he has not had a disparity between his experiences and behaviour. It wasn't always like that, but he managed to achieve it in recent years. He managed to do it by declaring: "When I do what I don't want, when I am not myself, I am making myself sick, so

I'll become congruent and take care of myself." He had to declare this to be able to not do what he doesn't want to and not be who he is not. It may seem selfish, but he encourages everyone in his life to do the same. I trust him deeply, look up to him, and soak up everything he says. I rarely disagree with him. I want to hear him, not me. I think he is brave and outspoken. I can sense that what he is offering, and what he himself practises, is not going to be easy for me because I tend to take everyone's desires seriously, except my own.

> Nowadays, I practise the same thing Ronnie did. I am a living example; otherwise, how could I encourage my patients to practice it.

I should read John Bowlby's book on attachment and separation.[14] "I imagine," Ronnie says, "what would happen to my daughter, Natasha, if I and my wife, the child's mother, would disappear. A complete disaster. Tragedy. Even if we reappeared again in a year and a half, the present attachment could never be renewed, it couldn't be restored." This is how Ronnie shows his sympathy, and that I shouldn't think nothing serious happened to me.

It all started with Ronnie phoning me late at night, saying there was a crisis, and could I go there to deal with the situation. They are calling for him, but it would be good training for me. OK, I'll go. I have to meet a woman named Anna, and she lives at Eaton Square. I wasn't aware, but this is one of London's most expensive areas. There is an elevator going up from the lobby. They let me in, and I can't believe my eyes. The apartment is incredibly glamorous and beautiful, like a museum. Alexander Calder's mobiles hang from the ceiling, and there is an original Miro on the wall. The husband releases movies and owns the rights to many famous films. The wife is taking part in a 40-day-long Arica training course.[15] They both attend these regularly, otherwise they don't spend much time together at home. They go around to exhibitions in Switzerland, Italy and Brussels. The husband reads John Lilly and Piotr Ouspensky. There are mandalas from India hanging on the walls. Anna speaks with a slight accent. She used to be an actress in Austria, which is how she became involved in an affair with her husband, who was married with a child at the time. It took a long time for him to get a divorce and now, 19 years later, Anna finds herself in the same situation as his then ex-wife. She found out that he has a mistress. Her husband sent a message, through a mutual friend, that he wanted a divorce and to marry his new love. Anna has two daughters with him, 12 and 9 years old. She is very tense: she clenches her fists, her face is very angry, but her aggression is turned against herself. She wants to commit suicide, to disappear from the face of the earth. As if it were her fault, as if she was defective: she feels shame. She has not eaten for four days, she finds food disgusting and she is just drinking rosehip tea. There is absolutely nothing she can use from what she learned at her Arica training, that method is not helpful in this situation. She is frightened of losing her husband. She is terrified of an independent, wealthy and beautiful woman taking him away from her. She is frightened of having to tell her daughters, and she is frightened of not being able to live independently, not being able to work to maintain herself. The only reason she has not killed herself is her two daughters.

The husband called her a useless waste of space during a fight, and he predicted she would end up in the gutter. He thinks she is a hopeless case. He hits her sometimes. Any time she is sick, he hates her. The guy is in New York City now, but he is coming back in four days. She is very angry with her husband, and he is also angry, irritated, and hates her for her spiritual search, even for Arica. Still, he reluctantly agrees for the three of us to sit down when he comes back, to discuss the situation. Anna thinks that despite all this, sex was good between them. When she was expecting, that was a terrible time. She used to throw up a lot, as if she had an allergy or illness. She had a caesarean section. It seems to me, her present situation is like the second stage of labour, no exit, no way out. She is squeezed from all sides. There is no escape route in any direction.

A few days later, the three of us sit down. Anna speaks about her fears for the future. She feels she is going to be scavenging from trash cans. She is revolted by poverty, as if her nightmare is becoming poor. Her husband sniggers. He is showing us that despite not yet making up his mind about the divorce, he has put a million pounds in Anna's bank account, and if they divorce, she would get another million. What is she terrified of? Billions of people have never seen this much money. He can't take Anna seriously, and I am also finding it difficult. I am poor, he should give me all that money.

It's Ronnie's strategy to send me to these places, as well as to Brixton, London's poorest area. I should always pay attention to human misery, he says, and that has nothing to do with one's financial situation. I shouldn't be distracted by the circumstances. Whether it is the greatest destitution or wealth, it doesn't matter. It doesn't make any difference if relationships are not working.

Leon's Zen seminar. An hour of zazen, then a Zen walk. We sing sutras. He suggests we read Norman O. Brown's *Love's Body* and the Zen instructions of Huang-po.

There is practically no difference between my regular journal and my dream journal because I don't remember my days or my nights. You have to practise Zen as if your life depended on it, and it probably does. Zen teaches you to have faith in yourself and not let anyone hurry you, push you here or there. Find your own centre, your own rhythm. The mind can't see the mind. If I am seeking Buddha externally, I neglect my own Buddha nature. We lost our heads when we found them on our necks. When you find your head on your neck, you are very pleased that you have never actually lost it. I notice all sorts of things because people tell me to be attentive to myself. For example, I always take something to read to the toilet. Why? To make sure I don't waste any time. Every minute is important, and if I lose something, I have to make up for it. I eat letters, and I am proud of the shit I defecate. And I am proud of being able to read in English. Both my shit and my reading are accomplishments. I am accomplished. Maybe I am reading so I don't have to pay attention to my shit. Then I notice that I don't urinate standing up, like a proper man. I always sit down. Why? Because I am too tall and my cock is too far from the toilet. I can't aim properly, and I don't want to mess up the toilet bowl. I don't want to clean it, and I don't want to leave it messy. It makes more sense to sit down. It occurs to me that my father didn't live with us, and when I saw my mother pee, she was always sitting down. I had a friend in Budapest, a watchmaker who was very tall, and he also always peed sitting down.

I feel I am making progress with my yoga practice. My body can do things it couldn't previously. It took two months. I can hold the asanas longer, and I am closer to the ideal poses. I am improving. Mina tells me about Iyengar, her master, who shouts and is rough.[16] It is difficult to work with him, but he is very good at loosening one's muscles. He had a student, a woman, and he stood on her thighs to help them open up. It is a little bit like Rolfing, painful but effective.[17] Mina cried a lot, there was a lot of pain and a lot of letting go. Mina's husband, Arthur, used to be a boxer, and somehow his neck sank in between his shoulders. His shoulders rose up to his ears. Yoga restored his neck, and he became a yoga instructor. But Arthur enjoys sadism. I trust everyone. I do a handstand and Arthur pushes his knee in my back, pulls back my shoulders. It's a burning feeling, and the muscles tear in my shoulders all over. I never allow him to touch me again. Mina never does anything like that. Arthur is from South Africa, which has an apartheid regime. He tells Ronnie he is moving back to South Africa. "Don't go back, you moron, you can't live in that place," Ronnie tells him. There is a farewell party, Ronnie is there. Then suddenly and unexpectedly, Ronnie jumps on Arthur like he is doing a rugby tackle and breaks both his legs. He has to go to the hospital, of course, and he doesn't go to South Africa.

Later, many years later, Arthur killed himself.

I am jealous that Ronnie likes Arthur so much. I am sure he wouldn't have broken my legs. The body is for bumping. I am going to see him for a session in the morning. He smiles at me. He has two front teeth missing. They were knocked out last night in a brawl in the pub. But he is not complaining, he is matter of fact about it. This is what the body is for. This is very alien to me. I am very careful with my body. My mother always treated me as if my body belonged to her, and I had to be very careful at all times. Once I fell off my scooter, and my knee and elbow were bleeding. I didn't feel any pain, but I was worried about her getting angry. When I had any problems with my body, she was angry as if I had broken one of her vases.

In a group called Practical Therapy, Ronnie is scaring most of the people. He walks around, and he is willing to fight with whoever is prepared to stand against him. You can do anything, nothing is forbidden, and you are free to fight. No holds barred. Who wants to fight with him? Well, not me, that's for sure, but Leon comes forward, and I nearly shit myself as these two set about fighting each other. Looks like they won't stop until one of them ends up dead. That's what men are like. I'd rather not be a man. I need no Rolfing, and I don't fight. Many women turn away or walk out of the group.

Later on, I used to wrestle with my patients a lot; if they preferred, we would start kneeling so neither of us would get hurt falling from a standing position, but when one of us said "stop", we would have to stop. I enjoyed that. I took part in a real fight only once on Kis Rókus Street, in Buda. Someone called me a Jew, and I didn't have the faintest idea what it meant. I was about six or seven, but I was overcome with rage. It had never happened to me in my life before. There are different colours of anger but I could only see red at the time. I jumped on this kid. He hit me square on and it hurt badly. I had a good friend, Tibi Sás, who had ginger hair and freckles, and everybody teased him. He was astonishing, he scratched, bit, kicked, and set about kids twice his size, so everyone was scared of him. But that wasn't my temperament. Árpi Korda was like a girl, a delicate pretty-boy, but when he got angry, he laid into people like anything. People feared him too, they left him alone. I wasn't anything like them but felt a lot of respect for them. Laing had street-smarts, he grew up in the Gorbals in Glasgow, a rough neighbourhood. I had a lot to learn.

I am working with Anna again. I am surprised that her husband is 50 and she is 42; they both look younger. Anna is particularly hurt by the affair because her husband got together with a woman, an acquaintance of Anna's, who is much younger than her and is very attractive. She feels defeated, like her light has been put out. She suddenly feels very old. Yesterday, she went to Wimpole Street, where traditional psychiatrists practise. She had a consultation with one and requested medication to treat her aching heart. She is terrified of losing control over her life, of her will becoming irrelevant. She is so petrified that she became obstinate; she is not eating, not sleeping and not meeting anyone.

She agonises over how to tell her children about the situation. She tells me to build her up. She asks me whether there is a risk of her committing suicide, what her chances are. I tell her, "How the fuck would I know, this is not an illness." She can do what she wants. The psychiatrist recommended that she go to a hospital and scared her with the increased statistical likeliness of children committing suicide if their mothers kill themselves. So, Anna is too scared to kill herself now. I speak with Ronnie about it at our supervision meeting. He can sense I don't like Anna asking for medication. He snaps at me. Who am I to judge her? I'll never have any idea how much she is hurting. If she wants to take medication, let her take medication. Well, we have cleared that up once and for all.

During our supervision meeting, Ronnie speaks about the many layers of wealth. Having grown up in a poor area of Glasgow, he was 30 when he first encountered wealth. My job is to get used to all sorts of environments, so I can pay attention to the person and not be distracted by things. Whether in dirty or glamorous surroundings, people's problems are the same. Jealousy and fear are the same in the rich and the poor. How much money should I ask for my time? Ronnie tells me to ask for as much as the person is used to. He has a go at me for asking too little from Anna. He tells me if I don't ask for as much as the person is used to, if I am content with the amount the plumber gets or even less, they won't take me seriously.

Anna's problem is a birth trauma; she needs to give birth to herself, now. She needs to separate herself from her husband. When the umbilical cord is cut, the child doesn't know where provisions will come from. They think they will starve to death until they realise how to get hold of the milk. We talk about Medard Boss, and according to him, every sexual perversion is a small gap in the wall one surrounds oneself with and contact is still possible through this gap. So, we shouldn't judge perversions negatively. The person may not allow anything else, so one has to start with that and widen the gap rather than bricking it up, judging or banning it.

There was a patient of Ronnie's who used to pay a lot of money to women to change his diapers. He peed and shat himself, and the woman had to gently clean him up and change him, so he could experience orgasm. Ronnie didn't put a stop to it at all. I didn't shake my head disapprovingly. After about two years, he lost all interest in this particular perversion. He now lives with a woman, and they have a little girl whom he likes very much. No one would suspect that he went through such a phase, that he indulged in this perversion. Ronnie had another male patient who put a green wig on the women he slept with, otherwise he was impotent. Later, I read Masud Khan[18], who says that perversions are due to the person not ever wanting to grieve. This is a kind of insurance policy: if his lover dies, no problem, he keeps the green wig and puts it on another woman. Women are interchangeable. Nothing personal. The wig is the important thing because it protects him from sex becoming intimate. Without the wig, he would be vulnerable. If someone leaves him or dies, he has to grieve for them, but no one will take away the green wig. Masud Khan speaks extensively about perversion. He is an expert on the topic.

Anna's husband is named Joe. I sit down with the two of them. He seems to me a rough and callous guy. He resents Anna for not being well. He doesn't want any problems, and he doesn't want people in their social circle to think badly of them. He is worried about how the children will cope with this. He wants me to cure Anna, so she can be strong, and happy about the divorce. He doesn't want Anna to have any doubts about the money. He will transfer so much money to her account, there will be no need for her to be anxious. He will look after her. He doesn't care, he says, who Anna sleeps with. He forgets that Anna is 42, and it is much easier for a 50-year-old man to have good sex with younger women than it is for an older woman to have sex with younger men. They are Jewish, so the family should stay together. They discuss that if they could have sex, freely, they could stay together. The children mustn't know anything about this.

It's Saturday evening. Anna turns up at my practice, all upset. She left her daughter's birthday party because she couldn't cope. Joe is there too, and she had to behave as if everything was normal. Anna is shaking. She is tense and closes her eyes. She realises that she is paralysed by not being able to make up her mind about staying with Joe, as if nothing had happened, or getting up the nerve to leave him. She doesn't want either, and she wants both. She utters this double bind and relaxes a bit. For 20 years, she had the whole Joe to herself, she thought she knew him, and now it turns out she only knew a small fraction of him. She asks me whether it was necessary to know the other person completely, or was this small percentage sufficient, could she continue with this small fraction. She is hoping for Joe to wake up, to show remorse, to apologise, to change, and for everything to be great like it used to be. But then she realises that what Joe feels and says is unimportant. She has to clear up something within herself.

With Steve, we talk about how he found the saboteur in himself. He says we should be prepared for the eventuality of him sabotaging our relationship as well. He feels I've placed him in a double bind: if he does sabotage, I am going to be right, and if he doesn't, then he can't do what he always does. He wants attention, but he is afraid of it, too. When his father paid attention to him, he controlled him at the same time. We settle on him moving the points around, to switch from "can't do" to "doesn't want to do", and that he should get rid of everything he *must* do. Nothing *must* be done.

On Sunday, Hugh Crawford's secretary, Doris, phones me to say that nearly everyone has left one of the shelters. They went to Wales for the weekend. Three brave ones remained: Doris, Zita and Eric. Doris doesn't know what to do with them, so she asks me to come over in the afternoon. Zita is at the cinema, so there is only Eric and Doris at home when I arrive. Doris is really anxious. She is frightened of Eric and can't talk to him properly. Eric is confident and collected, but every so often, he laughs without any apparent reason. It is difficult to follow what he says because he speaks in an abstract and hazy way. His eyes, hair and beard are dark brown, and he is a thin, sinewy chap. He keeps jumping up and striding around in circles. He gets behind my back and hits my shoulder with his fist a couple of times. He says he was angry with me, but he also says he hoped that he didn't hurt me.

We arm wrestle. It's better than him hitting me. He is so tense, he is thrown off balance and loses every time, although his strength matches mine. Doris is like an anxious mother. She makes tea, brings some food, and she is always on the go, getting something done. Zita returns home. Later, Hugh Crawford arrives, and I find myself in the middle of a family scene. Hugh is the father, Doris is the mother, and Eric and Zita are the children. Crawford is ruthless with Zita. He deals with Eric much more gently, even though Eric goes up to Zita twice to punch her. Crawford screams at Zita. He thinks her pretend weakness is tyrannical. He demands complete semantic precision. Eric, for example, says that Zita was controlling him. Zita says she didn't want to control him. Crawford screams at them that he didn't say "you were *trying* to control him," but that "you *were* controlling him." Zita says that Eric was sending vibrations with his hand, and it scared her. He was shooting energies into her. Crawford screams, "This is bullshit, madness, omnipotence, almightiness, and what kind of energies or vibrations could he put into you!" Zita says that she can't be in the same room with Eric. Crawford is so angry, he explodes: "I won't tolerate that in this house! That's a judgement! This house is not about that!"

Each shelter has its own character, depending on the leader and those who live there. Something like this could never happen in Ronnie's or Leon's house, but those who can cope in Hugh Crawford's house are benefited by it. He is always himself. He dominates like a king, but because he shows his emotions and is frank, whoever can cope with it, it does them good. If one doesn't like it, they can look for another house. Just as well, as there are many houses.

The next day, I talk about Hugh with Ronnie. Ronnie thinks Hugh doesn't believe women have consciousness, and that he is terribly pessimistic. Jutta doesn't even let Hugh enter their house. Ronnie thinks he is too much of a moralist. Ethics (universal, to do with how we treat each other, to do no harm) are fine, but morality (local, traditional, customary, habitual) is not. We also discuss Anna and Joe, who found a psychiatrist, but he isn't prepared to go to their house. They have to go and see him at his office. Ronnie thinks it is very important that patients are aware that the therapist can't be bought or manipulated. This psychiatrist feels safer at his office, but I am OK to go and see them if I am confident about my boundaries. The apartment can provide a wealth of information if I can look after myself, but if I can't, it's best to just work in my office. Ronnie warns me that it will be too easy just to blame Joe, and feel sorry for Anna. As Hugh calls Zita's weakness tyrannical, Anna is also trying to control Joe with hers.

A 23-year-old man comes to see Ronnie. I am also there. He is Julian. He came from the hospital, where he had electroshock treatment every three weeks to save him from sinking too far into what he calls "deep thinking". He was fired from his job two years ago, and then he thought deeply for three months. He didn't eat, he didn't get up from his bed, and he got bedsores. Those who knew him started panicking and arranged electroshock treatment for him. He says once he only thought about colours for 24 hours. Ronnie is very open and understanding. He accepts Julian's thesis. He doesn't consider him mad at all but he says that first there has to be preparations made for these things. You can't just get into them. He should learn to fast and read books about it. "If you need regression, then use it. Even if you become very thin, that's fine. If you end up in hospital, they will fatten you up with intravenous drips, instead of giving you electroshocks. Even that's not a big problem, but you need to be smart about it." Ronnie agrees with Julian completely. This thing needs to be thoroughly contemplated, even if it takes years. But he has to be careful. He has to do it without alarming, shocking, or outraging anyone. To become acceptable, it is helpful to have a therapist who is sympathetic. Getting an electroshock is like being hit in the head with a club, it gives you a concussion and eventually it stops all thinking. If he wants to think, he shouldn't allow himself to be constantly hit in the head. Julian says that he tried to attend therapy but he couldn't get up for morning appointments. According to Ronnie, there is, unfortunately, nowhere in England where he could go to be looked after. Regression is not tolerated. We agree that he will see me for late afternoon sessions, and one of the shelters may let him move in and stay there. They could possibly look after him.

A Greek woman comes. She is a psychologist, translating Ronnie's books into Greek. She says in Greece, psychiatry is very conservative and reactionary. Ronnie explains that he is not into anti-psychiatry, he has no illusions about being original, and he doesn't hope to change the world. The woman is married with two children, she lives in Greece, and she has a cousin diagnosed with catatonic schizophrenia. She would like this cousin to meet Ronnie. Ronnie says he is prepared to meet him, at least once. He will introduce him to the Philadelphia Association, and he can have a look around, but Ronnie can't promise anything else. He is always very careful not to promise anything he is not sure about. But the cousin should come, somebody should accompany him to London, and someone should be available to take him back home if he doesn't want to stay in London. He is very rational. To me, he also said, "we will see." He didn't promise anything. At most, his encouragement sounded like, "Things should work out alright."

I begin reading *The Trauma of Birth*, by Otto Rank.[19] The first chapter is on the situation of analysis. In my therapy with Ronnie, the seed, the essence of the analytic process is to repeat one's separation from the mother, but more successfully, less painfully, this time. According to Winnicott, anger is good. If someone, a child or patient is angry, that's good because it means they still have hope for change. Once a child loses faith that change is possible, there is no anger. They cease wanting anything. This is early depression, or absolute hopelessness, helplessness. Originally, crying was probably caused by pain or hunger after birth. Later, when the source of crying is anger, fear, or sadness, then pain, trouble or discomfort are already familiar. It either was, or it is, coming. At this point, crying shows that the child has ideas, fears and memories. Sadness is a sense of responsibility for one's environment. It happens when a child thinks that they made a mess of something, or that they broke something. I discuss my limited range of emotions with Ronnie. He says it could be the result of fashion or culture, either familial or national. I would have turned out differently if I had been born in Italy. It is also possible, however, that I am trying to avoid pain, which comes with a whole spectrum of emotions. Joy has its flip side; it comes with pain. "How great" has its "how grim". But I avoid everything if I want to avoid pain. Ronnie recites Catullus: "I hate and I love. Why I do this, perhaps you ask. I know not, but I feel it happening, and I am tortured."[20] We talk about how it was so important for my mother to potty-train me very early. She was constantly scrubbing me and she wanted me to be obedient. My mother made my clothes and she used to always iron everything I wore. I wasn't allowed to be muddy, and I had clean white shoes. Ronnie is looking at me and says that, as he sees me now, he thinks I have rebelled. My present appearance is a reaction. My hair is shaggy, but so is his. Jutta, his wife, is begging him to stop all this revolution. Of course, European intellectuals tend to be scruffy. A shame, I say, but for him it is more important how his body feels in the clothes than how the clothes look. This is typical of my discussions with Ronnie: even the smallest things are important, and he is always personal, not abstract.

I meet John Heaton again, and he appears to be happy to see me this time. He is not attacking me. He allows me to take part in his seminar for Philadelphia Association therapists. He lets me be part of the big group, and I learn about Edmund Husserl with him. I am very happy to be able to work with Laing, Huxley, and Heaton.

I am reading Winnicott. He says adults have a hard time giving in to the excitement they could experience in each other's company, and he thinks it originates from their mother being frightened of her baby's appetite, hunger, and desire. If the mother becomes scared when she gives the baby her breast, the baby, as they grow up, will think that the world will be afraid of their appetite. Someone whose mother was afraid that they would devour her breast is going to become frightened of an exciting hunger or an exciting desire. It will tarnish the adult's joie de vivre, sexuality and relationship with food.[21]

Francis is forty minutes late for his seminar. We play drums while waiting. He speaks about tantrums, fits of temper or rage, and how these are always about honour. If the sense of "I am me" or the awakening to this fact comes too early, the restrictions usually placed on children are terribly uncomfortable and restrictive for said children. Children whose awakening comes later tend to have an easier childhood. Standing up for myself is a very lonely undertaking. Honour is sometimes so important that it leads to violence. Only blood can wash away the insult. "Hungarians," says Francis, "were famous for having a code of honour that demanded they kill themselves within 24 hours if they couldn't pay their gambling debts by the designated deadline." Society's most dangerous addiction is gambling; one might gamble away all their possessions, their spouse, their house, everything. Rockefeller is like a tribal chief, Francis tells us, he distributes his money in return for loyalty. We discuss how desire turns into wilfulness and demands. We talk about Stanislavski, who trained actors' willpower.[22] Liza Minnelli can only sing when she is liberated from all resentment. If one gives their everything to whatever they are doing then they have to become unencumbered by any hard feelings and grudges. Anger narrows one's consciousness, one's spirit. When Liza sings, she opens up completely. You can't do that if you are harbouring some resentment. One may wake up to the fact that life is bullshit, and smart people therefore kill themselves – that is what the ancient Greeks used to say – and it is possible to carry on living after one no longer wants to. So, life can be an art. One should live as one wants to, in the style one wishes to. That is why it's worth living even when one no longer wants to. There are very few people – Ronnie is one of them – who can awaken others' resolve, because those who just want to want don't really want. But Ronnie has this magic or witchcraft that awakens people's real resolve. Francis talks about how drinking or smoking alone is not good. It will make one ill and isolated. It is an offence or a sin. But doing the same thing in a group may become togetherness and communion. Laing called it *conviviality*. So, he doesn't think marijuana is bad if it is smoked in a gathering, or if it is passed around from one person to the next. No one smokes a whole joint when it is shared. Like Scottish people, who gather in the evenings at a cèilidh to sing, recite poetry and pass around the whiskey, the mood heightens as they spend time together.[23] The Yiddish word *chutzpah* often refers to tongue-in-cheek audacity, brazenness, cockiness when someone is involved in something shitty but turns it into gold. The classic example is someone kills their father and mother and then asks the court for leniency on the basis of being an orphan. I steal, someone finds out, and I say that only idiots don't steal, everyone else does. There is an old saying from England and the USA: "Hungarians are the only people who can go into a revolving door behind you, and come out of it in front of you." Well, that's *chutzpah*. To create something good from a bad thing or action, something I can be proud of rather than being embarrassed by. If I have *chutzpah*, I never have to feel embarrassed. Whoever tries to accuse or condemn me will end up feeling like an idiot. It gives you a huge sense of self-confidence. Honour is always relative, often amoral, and there are cultures where honour and truthfulness are not linked. I pay for everyone's round in the pub even if I don't have a penny to my name. I pretend to be rich and I designate it a matter of honour. There is often competition in honour. At one time, Hungarians were famous for committing suicide rather than owing money to someone. Honour can be fatal sometimes.

At Haya Oakley's seminar, we discuss Joseph from the Bible, who was the first dream-reader. Consciousness is always consciousness of something, says Oakley. There is no empty consciousness. According to Heidegger, she tells us, dreams are interesting and unlike reality because in dreams the correlation of time and space is different. Medard Boss thinks "I am having a dream" is not accurate, not true; even "I am dreaming" is inaccurate. "Someone is dreaming me" is the actual truth. This is a real phenomenological description.

On October 25th, 1974, I attend Ronnie's seminar. He is speaking about beginnings, where it starts, biologically and psychologically. One's life starts at birth, not conception. This was the accepted view when he was a medical student. For quite a long time, foetuses and babies weren't considered sentient beings. But for Ronnie, it has always been obvious that life starts at conception. Sometimes science doesn't recognise things, although they are evident. Ronnie worked with John Bowlby in the Tavistock

Clinic, and for Bowlby, it was clear that a child who loses their mother must suffer deeply negative consequences. This wasn't accepted without evidence. He had to prove it. Ronnie talked with Winnicott about mythology being a projection of prenatal life. This is another thing that was obvious to Winnicott and Ronnie, yet scientific psychology still doesn't take it seriously. Francis Mott wrote a lot about one's experiences in the womb.[24] He says every human is one cell in the beginning then they start to divide, becoming a duality, then a trinity, and this trinity remains: foetus, placenta and umbilical cord. When the father's and mother's chromosomes unite and the chromosome that is you comes into existence, you live as a tiny zygote for a while. A lot of symbols become meaningful in this way. The tree of life, for example, gains relevance when we understand that the placenta, with its web of veins, looks like a tree. We are the fruit on the tree, we are hanging on the tree and we are ripening and falling off. *Placenta* means "cake" in Latin. This is the origin of the birthday "cake", celebrating birth; we used to eat the placenta. Mott talks about how the veins are also very interesting; every vein divides into two branches, then divides again, and there are millions of branches in the placenta. Inside the umbilical cord, two arteries twist around the red vein. This, in itself, looks like a caduceus or a kerykeion, the staff with two serpents entwined around it, which is the symbol of Hermes. The placenta, which connects the mother and the foetus, has an overall surface area of about five square meters. It is also important to know, he thinks, that when we are born and the cord is cut, in actuality part of the child is cut off since the placenta, the cord and the child are one unit. So, the placenta belongs to the child, not the mother.

In other words, unless they wait for the cord to dry off naturally, an amputation is performed. Mott says that as after any amputation, the memory of the limb is like a phantom limb and it stays behind in the consciousness. In our brains, there is a map of the placenta and the umbilical cord. Then it emerges in mythology and fairy tales in the form of sky-high trees and serpents. This is mind-blowing! The newborn projects this map of consciousness on their mother's breast and kneads their mother with their feet. This creates an experience similar to the womb and this movement stimulates the mother's body, the hormones for the milk let-down reflex. The system is perfect. You could turn it into biological theology. The father's sperm and the mother's ova unite into one, into everybody's source. This is the origin, the genesis, and this could be the beginning of biological theology.

Ronnie speaks about this as well, but it is important for us to know, and to note, that the first cell already finds itself in a given environment in the fallopian tube. There is no organism without an environment. It seems that, somehow, with these early encounters, the quality of the environment we find ourselves in – whether it is positive, negative or zero, or in other words, whether it is inimical and averse or neutral or accepting and joyful – continues to resonate within us. It is as if our relationship with, our expectations of, our environment has been fixed. The recent science of epigenetics might account for this. Then we have this mythological motif, the first parents losing or wanting to lose their child. They place him in a basket, like Moses, and let him float off on the river. Then a new mother or a new set of parents come and they adopt him. They bring him up. Otto Rank believes the reason for this archetypal motif is people not wishing to accept that their parents are their real parents. One creates a hopeful fantasy that these are just one's adoptive parents and somewhere out there exist one's good and highly intelligent real parents. Francis thinks this motif also originated from the womb. The first parents are the memory of conception, the basket is the shape of the morula or blastula, the river is the fallopian tube where one sails down to reach the shore, to embed oneself where one can develop peacefully.[25] After embedding, only the embedded blastula survives. This is the origin of the religious ideas that we have to die in order to live because those who are not buried cannot live. All these steps are so deeply ingrained in us that anything we ever embark on in life, relationships, books, anything, follows this same pattern. Anywhere we go, the expectation of emotion, whether it is fear or joy, originates from this. Then, when we are born, that is the third adoption. The danger is ever-present: maybe we can't embed, maybe we can't be born. It is always uncertain whether we can survive the trials and tribulations. At the age of 20, I, for example, was afraid to enter a restaurant. I was scared of everyone looking at me and sometimes I felt it would be better not to go in. And if I did happen to go in, then three minutes later, I was staring at those who had just arrived. I was an insider by then, not an outsider any more. Perhaps it wasn't easy for me to enter my mother's endometrium. At the start of embryonic existence, there is no rhythm because there is no heart. Every rhythm comes from the outside. My own rhythm starts when my heart starts beating. Embedding can be simultaneously very attractive and very frightening. There are some people, and this sometimes borders on insanity, who are constantly terrified of their surroundings. This primary anxiety doesn't go away because one cannot live without an environment. These people are prescribed medication because doctors don't know how to deal with such fears. Sometimes, if the person goes into regression, either through hypnosis or with a tolerant therapist, they can go back and turn off the alarms. There are some who have this sense of their consciousness being like a sponge and it is saturated with trepidation or joy. But it all feels like a sphere: dread and happiness come from all directions. That's why Francis believes it to be the memory of the blastula.

According to Victor Tausk and Nándor Fodor, the placenta may be conceptualised as the twin I am making love to, because with each heartbeat I ejaculate into him and he ejaculates into me.[26] There is a movement of fluids between two huge things. This is the origin of Isis and Osiris, the divine amorous couple who were already lovers in Nut's (the sky goddess's) womb. If the bodily sensation of fear comes from all directions, then it is an earlier memory than that of fear coming from one direction (fear of being poisoned, for instance). There is another crucial duality: we feel safe in the womb, but after a certain amount of time, our territory becomes too constricted. The more we grow, the more it turns into a prison. Stanislav Grof believes there is "bliss inside," which, as our world becomes more constricted, is followed by a sense of "no exit," which we become released from by a "bloody battle" to achieve the sense of "bliss outside".[27] Every outside becomes inside and every safety turns into a prison.

There are some people in some of the shelters who eat from the floor and shit on the floor. Ronnie believes when one goes into regression, one goes back to the womb, one eats and evacuates there, and the floor is the placenta. This is, of course, just a metaphor because science can't explain how one could remember without a nervous system, so it is impossible to prove scientifically. Yet it is essential to think about this because if the argument is even a little bit sound in terms of scientific rationale, then we have to take very good care of mothers and their unborn babies. Ronnie thinks we have to let go of the idea that we can do anything with newborns because they won't remember anything anyway. Thus, if there is prenatal and perinatal memory, there must be psychology also. There are common memories and experiences that speak in the language of symbols, in the language before words. Lucifer is science lacking love.

A young woman comes to see me. She is the daughter of a psychiatrist friend and says things like "I am too tired to talk", "You can't know me, and you can't understand me at all when I say something." She says "you confuse me, you hurt me, you don't help me." She doesn't look at me and she avoids my eyes. We are not getting anywhere. I invite her to have dinner at my home, with my family, but she says she is too distressed to eat. Then she stays anyway and devours everything we have with an excellent appetite. I tell her we are finished now because we must leave. We have tickets for a ballet performance. But she takes it that we were trying to get rid of her. She doesn't move. She is crying. We leave her sitting outside on the common stairs. She phones the next day to tell me she doesn't trust me. I ask Ronnie what he thinks. He says that by inviting her to eat with the family, I stirred up all sorts of fantasies, which created further separation anxieties. I should only do this if I am ready to go deeply into dealing with these anxieties. Once or twice, he also allowed some people to stay with him but then he was determined to accept this closeness for an extended period. If I am not prepared to do that, then I should remain within the standard boundaries of therapy.

We also spoke about how it was good to have a place where one can scream, shout, and cry. In a soundproofed room, for example, or if that is not available, one could go out to a big park and scream there at dawn. Ronnie agrees with me that the woman backed herself into a corner and now she can't come out. She is the living reminder to all of us, to her parents, to me, to everyone, that we failed. She sacrifices her own life to make sure everyone has a miserable time because of her. Ronnie says sometimes I express a similarly stubborn mechanism. When I don't tell him about my dreams and thoughts, when I don't share everything with him, then he has this same feeling of having failed. We talk about touch. When he was a child, he had small blisters on his body, especially on his hands and legs. They hurt and itched, so he was very careful about touch. He encourages me to be very attentive to my needs, to what I want to see, hear, taste, touch and smell. In every relationship, with every person, we have these thoughts and desires, and he thinks it is important that one know what one wants to experience through one's senses, and what one doesn't want to experience. He contemplates whether I am able to read other people's signals sensitively enough and how close can I get to them. If I am too scared of someone pushing me away, he says, then I will never be able to find out what is around me in the world. If I am not worried about loss, being pushed away, being rejected or excluded, then I can allow myself to be spontaneous. I feel helpless more than anything else, I tell him. That's fine, he replies. Why do I think that others don't think of themselves as clumsy? According to Winnicott,[28] there is a natural process, already present with babies, related to their mother's breast. It is the cruel (loveless) desire for nourishment, which is the source of the aggressive attack, that then turns into a feeling of guilt. This sets off the sense of "I'll take care of you", followed by sadness, and the desire to rectify the relationship, to build or to give. After becoming anxious and careful, we become upset that the other person is not indestructible. You can observe this in small babies: first they grab the breast as if it belonged to them, but then they realise that the mother's face and her breast are one, and they are frightened. Then comes guilt, especially when they bite the mother and the mother cries out. Winnicott calls this process "the birth of ruth" – the path from ruthlessness to ruth, which is an old English word for love.

Ronnie tells me to pay attention to my thoughts to discover the modus operandi.[29] Where do thoughts come from? From the right and behind or from the left and front? He thinks thoughts come from different directions. I should observe what I do with them. Do I push them aside, push them to the back, push them down, disperse them, destroy them, or do I do something else? Free association is to avoid censorship. It's a question of deciding to do it. Even when I feel ashamed, I still talk about everything, including even my struggle with this censorship. This is the "psychoanalytic contract" Freud required of his patients.

I met up with Anna and her husband this evening. The Mexican psychiatrist, Roberto, was also there. Anna and Joe think this is what is required. Roberto calls me the next day to tell me that he thinks Anna is impulsive and impotent, and that was the source of her confusion. And that Joe is omnipotent and narcissistic. Since Anna is offended and ambivalent, she can't support Joe, and her malice and terrible anxiety provokes reserve and closing up. The more anxiety she feels, the more Joe becomes reserved. And, Anna confuses Joe with her father. He may prescribe a mild tranquiliser to Anna and I should continue therapy with her and Joe.

Sometimes Winnicott seems like a male chauvinist, but I still find lots of exciting ideas in his work. He thinks in terms of a traditional family set-up, with the father as head of the family and the mother as secondary. I find it disturbing but I usually read – sometimes even difficult texts, like Lacan – as if I were swimming in it. If I don't agree with something or I don't under-stand something, I just swim through it and concern myself with the things I find interesting. This is how I keep swimming around in Winnicott's, Lacan's and Laing's work. Of course, they have to remain authentic for this and I must regularly find things that grab my attention. If I didn't find anything, I would stop reading them. There are very few writers whose books I keep returning to. Books by Thomas Szász or Erich Fromm are stimulating but I don't return to them. I've finished them. But it is impossible for me to finish Winnicott's, Lacan's, Laing's or Bion's books.

William Blake, Sigmund Freud, Masud Khan, Sándor Ferenczi, Marion Milner, Alan Watts, Swami Vivekananda, Stanislav Grof, Slavoj Žižek and Jacques Lacan – I never feel I have fin-ished reading their books.

I go to a party in the afternoon, and Ronnie and Francis are there. I just stare in amazement as Ronnie lets his son, Adam, kick and hit his back as hard as he wants. He sits on the ground, protects his kidneys with his arms, and Adam sets about him. He is about eight. I am surprised.

Years later, I tried this with my kids, Marcel and Soma. They were delighted to have a fight with me like this. They didn't hurt me. They were happy I could survive their aggression.

I observe people just letting their kids wander around freely at the party. No one puts them to sleep. When they get exhausted, they fall asleep somewhere on a carpet or a sofa. Ronnie tells us about the time he served as an officer in the British army. He was leading a detachment of soldiers who were marching towards a wall. He got lost in his thoughts for a moment, and when he looked up, he could see them marching into the wall. He said "halt" at the last second. Well, he doesn't want his kids to be obedient because obedience reminds him of this: the idiots marching into the wall.

I ask Ronnie if I can attend his seminars on Mondays. There are only six students, and I am the seventh because he lets me come. He is incredibly accepting. He obviously likes me. It scares me, but I am happy about it at the same time. I am worried he appreciates me more than I deserve it. When he realises who I am, he is going to drop me and that is going to hurt a lot. I tell him about this worry, but he just smiles.

I quiz Ronnie about the American trend of personality development and self-growth. He says there are two kinds of growth, referring to perinatal things again. There is cell division without differentiation, the blastula. The morula is just reproducing but there is no differentiation. The same thing repeats itself over and over again. This kind of growth is like people shopping for experiences, later on. After embedding, a different kind of growth starts called cellular differentiation. Some cells will become bones, some skin and some organs. Such growth only happens by itself and only in certain situations. Self-development groups only facilitate the first kind of growth because people don't digest their experiences, they just place more and more things in their basket.

We talk about geometric shapes like squares and circles. Do they have a psychological or mythological manifestation? In hypnosis, or in an altered state of consciousness, I have very different emotions spring up when I think of a square than when I think about a circle, even the colours are different. We meander around to Kronos, who devoured his children. So, after Rhea gave birth to Zeus, she hid him and handed Kronos a stone wrapped in swaddling clothes, saying that was his child. Kronos was an idiot who didn't notice anything amiss, so he promptly swallowed the stone. Thus, Zeus and Rhea survived and Kronos was finally killed by his own son, as foretold by the prophecy.

Ronnie tells me it is very important to learn some skill that can help one towards experiencing communion. Communion, unity and community don't just happen by themselves. There has to be an effort. One has to learn certain things necessary to achieve it; for example, singing, playing instruments, dancing or martial arts. In other words, things we can do together, things that merge us into one entity. After achieving a certain level of competence, you become one with the action, the performer becomes one with the performance. This is the actual flow, the beatitude (supreme happiness) of experiencing oneself as a small part of something big.

My talks with Ronnie often start disastrously and I feel clumsy. I am embarrassed because I can't dance, play music or do judo well. Each time we talk, I have to work my way through shame, but I long for the inspiration, so I don't avoid these challenges. I sing a lot, which is a big thing for me because my first-grade teacher told me to stand among the children in the choir but not to sing, to just mouth the words because I was "tone-deaf" and I sang off-key. I believed her, but Ronnie says anyone can learn to sing in tune. It's just a question of practice. He gives me a tuning fork. I have to hit it on my head and practise by humming the pure note. Then two minutes silence and hum again, correcting myself with the tuning fork if necessary. When I can hum the pure note even after half an hour or an hour, then I am not singing off-key any more. We have opened the door closed by that stupid teacher.

It's easy to shoo away the other person by saying that they have some deficiency. If they are dyslexic or tone-deaf, we don't need to have anything to do with them. We don't need to take them seriously because that is often a lot easier than taking an interest, spending the time, and carefully and gently finding the personalised method for them. It is easier to pay attention to those who are already doing what we want them to do because we need a lot of patience for those who can't do it yet. Oliver Sacks has enormous amounts of patience for his patients.[30] Time is required, but they say there is no time. Those who speak about "slow medicine", like Victoria Sweet,[31] have worked out that, in the long run, we save money by curing people slowly and patiently. Impatience is very expensive.

Ronnie has a dream of a Texan millionaire donating a huge amount of money to build a hospital that would be the first of its kind. He dreams about a five-star hotel with a sauna, a pool, a helipad and an airport. It would be at the beach, away from the city, with modern state-of-the-art technology, a laboratory, modern management, 24-hour service, nurses, doctors, chefs and everything that's necessary. Due to a lack of money, the shelters are bare, dirty and modest; it would be great if they could provide much better facilities. If the present is too much for someone because the past demands to be dealt with, if they need regression, if they can't look after and maintain themself, that is despicable in a capitalist civilisation and competitive society. If you are finding it hard to cope with life, then, well, get your act together. Ronnie wants to create a place where one can have a breakdown without having to feel ashamed about it. Madness is synonymous with wilfulness. Regression is a state of consciousness one can slip into and even get stuck there. It's a dimension: moving left, I feel younger and younger, moving right, I feel older and older. The journey to the right is progression, travelling to the left is regression. Hypnosis can move you one way or the other and so can certain drugs. Illness always takes you to the left, to dependence. On the left, you can crawl all the way back to conception, and on the right, to the present moment. When someone acts like a child, they may be in regression or they may be wilfully manipulating you. Only my

146

own emotions can give me a clue about who was doing what. If my heart opens easily and I am happy to mother the other person, then they are probably in regression. If I want to shake them angrily and to scream at them to stop it, then they are just having a tantrum. Laing dreams of this shelter as an elegant and expensive place, and this could show the world how valuable those are who live there. The world might even feel jealous/envious instead of pitying the patients. In a hospital, there should be real hospitality. And yes, there should be an optional padded room in this shelter. One can check in there if one wants to scream and kick the walls. One could let it all out and wouldn't have to control oneself. This hospital, or shelter, is not a punishment. One can request a stay there to regress peacefully.

I am reading Francis's book about the Urubu. Well, these people are cannibals. They organise ritual executions. Their mythology of creation is full of outlandish stories. It's very interesting. For example, first, their bodies had only one hole, their mouth, and they used it for eating and then vomiting to discard the waste. But their gods found this disgusting, so the chief god placed them on his knees one by one, and with a sharp stick pierced a hole in their arse. And men originally didn't have cocks. The whole tribe only had one cock that lived in the earth and the women kept it a secret. They didn't tell the men. The women used to go to the forest, hit the earth three times, the cock emerged, and then the women sat on it and had a fabulous time. But a Urubu man once hid and saw what the women did. He went to the forest at night, hit the earth three times, and when the cock emerged, he cut it down. He wanted to fix it onto himself, but he couldn't. Then he realised he could use sticky paste. When the other men came, he gave them each a piece, and that's how all men have their own cocks now. They did this to draw the women to themselves. But sometimes, the glued-on cock got stuck inside a woman or broke off.

Francis believes our whole civilisation feels ashamed. We constantly pollute our environment and despite making excuses, we know we shouldn't. We are ashamed: we are ashamed of Hitler, of allowing families to fall apart, of Vietnam, and of treating the younger generation badly. If a civilisation or an individual lives in shame for an extended period, they will perish, at least in spirit. We drive each other to madness with this double bind. According to Gilles Deleuze and Félix Guattari, schizophrenia is a consequence of capitalism.[32] We sink into the earth in shame. The opposite of shame is honesty, integrity and honour: all a result of duties well- fulfilled. Shame arises from neglecting and/or ignoring these duties. The more one complains, the more one will be belittled and humiliated by those around one. If one doesn't want to be humiliated, one shouldn't complain. The Philadelphia Association and this whole thing around Ronnie is about honour and shame. The members have an agreement. What is shameful in this company may not be shameful elsewhere, and what is honourable here may not be respected elsewhere. Whatever such-and-such is proud of in their life or in their work, I wouldn't be proud of; and whatever I am proud of, they would be ashamed of. It is interesting to look at things from this perspective. Instead of pondering who is right and who is wrong, we could reflect on where we belong. We belong to different tribes and families. We have different things to feel ashamed of and different things that make us proud. The difficulty is, of course, when the other tribe is in power and starts punishing what my tribe is proud of. When we have disagreements, the only way to cooperate is by explicitly stating everything, not hiding anything and not complaining about each other in secret. A good discussion between people of different views consists in everyone laying all their cards on the table, everything that was tucked away previously.

A community that has crumbled into pieces can only heal if the members rediscover and relearn appreciating each other and being honest with each other. Honour and trust need to be reborn.

Marriage may be a lockup in a global lunatic asylum, but it may be a shelter, too. It is crucial to recognise that human life consists of several strata, and they all work together. A lot of people are confused or lose their bearings because their lives are full of double binds. I feel I am cursed if I turn right, but if I turn left, that always leads to a disaster. There is no good direction. A pure sense of determination may sometimes help one escape this predicament. Zazen, samurai, Freud, and Arthur Schopenhauer all say that our particular decision doesn't matter. It doesn't matter whether we turn left or right, we just have to decide to want it. Then there is no double bind. One has to want and act. The outcome doesn't have to be perfect. It is important to note that one can distinguish between what is possible to want and what cannot be wanted. I can't change my emotions, so that cannot be wanted. If I don't want to feel what I am feeling, I'll become sad. Willpower doesn't change emotions. If you want to change your emotions, you need to act differently. This is what they believe at the Palo Alto Mental Research Institute,[33] and this is the opinion of Schopenhauer, who went for a walk at 2 o'clock every afternoon. He went regardless of rain or wind. He did this for many years, and this action must have influenced how he felt. It may be a discipline, a sports car, a university or a language we learn, but whatever we give ourselves to transforms us when we come out the other side.

For determination, it is necessary to be continuously alert. If we don't concentrate our attention, there is no willpower. If we actually pay attention to what we have decided, then others' opinions are irrelevant. It is a lie or mystification to say that one action leads to another. I have to do this *because* I have done that is not the case. Every moment is critical. I have to pay attention and use my willpower to be resolute. I have to wake up to the fact that I am alone and I am responsible for everything. Once I realise this, I have to sacrifice my isolated self, I have to dedicate the individual self (and it is not easy in our society) to the universe, to the community. But sometimes, the difference between being mad and having a good life depends on whether I can dedicate myself to some greater purpose. One cannot know anything without action. There is no abstract knowledge. Only doing leads to knowing. There is no need to compete for originality. One can learn tradition and a good life wherever one serves. The purpose of life is service. None of us is responsible for our origins, but we are accountable for the continued flow of the process that we entered. We shouldn't stop the flow of life in ourselves because we are responsible for its continued flow.

Francis says we can't live outside society, but if society is destroying itself, then the individual has to decide that they don't want to kill themselves. They don't want to die with the society, so they have to distance themself from it. If we don't know what is worth fighting for and dying for, then we naturally don't know what is worth living for. The worst thing is to die before one dies. I am alive as long as I have desires and hopes. As long as I am curious, I can enjoy the moment. Once I give these up, once I am just waiting for it all to end, I am not alive any more. No matter how much Francis criticises Ronnie, he still says we were very fortunate to have a master living among us. (Francis is constantly grumbling, but I think he likes and respects Ronnie. He criticises him here and there, if for nothing else, just so he doesn't feel inferior.) He considers Ronnie a master and he believes the reason Ronnie's behaviour is sometimes unacceptable, and one actually feels embarrassed by it, is just so he doesn't become a role model. Ronnie doesn't want to become an ideal. He is often drunk. He doesn't talk to anyone. He turns his back on everyone at parties and just plays the piano. If you expect him to keep your one-to-one discussions with him private, you are in for a big surprise when he publicises everything you told him. He doesn't keep secrets. You can't idolise him, that's for sure.

Intelligence is a social phenomenon. You need a lot of people to be intelligent. Intelligence emerges in a communication network. You can't be intelligent on your own. One has to consecrate one's life so that it is not just mundane but also sacred. How do you find what is sacred in you? Give yourself up to the following exercise: practice taking notice of what you pay attention to, and notice where your attention moves by itself when you are not deliberately concentrating on something. What is beyond our will is our sacred bit. There is no point in living if you don't give yourself to something, give of yourself. As a therapist, especially, one can't get away without it. We can't let ourselves slip into cowardice. Because you do need courage for this. If you allow yourself to slip into cowardice, you will have to pay the price of endless resentment, which leads to an uprising, a revolution. One wants to kill whatever forced one to become a coward and to cower. *Circulus vitiosus.*[34] According to Francis, good therapy is when the therapist makes an alliance with their patient as if they were their assistant. A professional doesn't hide anything. They deal with everything openly. It is always a pleasure to meet professionals.

I am at Haya Oakley's seminar. She is talking about a 29-year-old man, Collin. He had a breakdown at 19 and he was stuck in catatonic immobility. He attended Haya's therapy three times a week, and for three years, he didn't say a word during the fifty-minute sessions. Even later on, there was at least thirty minutes of silence during their sessions. He was a twin, born after his brother. After the first boy was born, he remained in the womb for at least another twelve hours. He had to be born, but he wasn't ready yet. He was immature, and he had no nails. To this day, he feels as though he hasn't been born, and his mother also says it's as if she hadn't given birth to him.

Every time Collin sits down, he feels anxious, so he paces up and down constantly, as if he were floating in space, he says. A few days ago, Haya showed him a picture of twins, and he went home, found a picture of himself and his twin brother and started to regress. His mother was there, and he fiercely attacked her. He screamed at her, and the woman wasn't strong enough to deal with the situation. There was a huge commotion, and they ended up being thrown out of their apartment. Collin's mother asked for her son to be accepted in one of the shelters, where he had spent time previously. So, Collin moved in, and somehow Mary Barnes ended up taking him under her wing. She encouraged him to wet his bed because it's really so much fun. Collin took possession of his room by throwing all the furniture out the window and down the stairs when he moved in. He created a new womb for himself. It wasn't easy with him. He kept breaking the windows. Somehow, he realised that the noise of the shattering glass makes everyone suddenly pay attention to him. Now, when he breaks something, he laughs and someone brings him some food to eat. He has been living in the shelter for a month, and his mother is furious about the whole thing. Haya thinks that for this guy to come alive, he has to kill his mother, hopefully only metaphorically and not literally. She is asking us to take care of him. We will need fourteen people, taking turns looking after him all day and all night. I volunteer, although I am scared. On the first day, I hardly dare enter his room. We have meetings where we discuss Collin, among other things. Someone suggests that we don't replace the glass when he breaks it the next time because it costs a lot of money. We should let him be cold.

Ronnie makes some calculations. It is cheaper to constantly replace the windows than to give medication, so let him carry on breaking it as long as he needs to. Collin is only prepared to eat the food that is placed on the floor, but that's where he defecates as well. We don't hurry him. We talk about how the floor is the placenta, and he needs the time he didn't get when he had to be born prematurely. But I can't deny it, we are looking forward to him stopping.

I am reading Carl Jung. I got an unpublished manuscript about dreams from somewhere. I have always been really interested in dreams. Jung says that as he got older, he became more and more adept at reading dreams, but simultaneously, his dreams became more and more complicated, so he found them ever difficult to read.[35] His dreamer is always smarter than his dream reader. He could only read others' dreams, never, without help, his own.

Winnicott notes. A year ago, when I worked with children in Vancouver, these notes would have been very useful. The section about children living with stress is equally true for children living in war zones and for children living in peace but with quarrels, fighting and aggression disrupting their families. An exciting notion is that children who settle easily in school, who separate themselves easily from the home environment, presumably had a pleasant experience when their mother weaned them. Scientific attitudes to human nature allow us to remain ignorant without having to be fearful. Science only really controls fear without actually taking us closer to understanding human nature. Thus, it regenerates itself because we need to create newer and newer theories to cover over what we don't know. According to Winnicott, good psychoanalysis means creating conditions for the patient to feel and think freely. In this freedom, they will sooner or later come across their own problematic bits. They will meet portions of themself that are not straightforward. So, in their relationship with their therapist, they will show the traumas that made their life difficult. The traumas that created afflictions they are too scared to approach on their own. So Winnicott believes that the patient was suffering because they had got stuck at a certain point. It is as if the trauma nailed them down somewhere, and they stopped growing at that point. Good therapy means the patient and the therapist remove the nail together, enabling the patient to carry on in their journey.

I visualise this as Marcel Duchamp's painting *Nude Descending a Staircase*. The woman's breasts are already at the bottom, her bum is still at the top, and she is stretched out like an accordion. This is how the patient exists. In therapy, their front stops, we wait for their back to catch up and join the rest, and then they can move forward as one unit. Once a particular tension ceases, it is easier to be in the present, and it is rarer for the past to crop up. Nothing can be replaced. We have to mourn what we lost, and we can delight in relief.

There is no such thing as a baby on their own. Only a baby with someone else, because the baby can't survive on their own. So, a baby is always part of a relationship. There is only a baby-in-relationship. Whatever is important when we are taking care of a baby is also important in therapy: can we rely on the caretaker? We need trust and confidence that we can rely on the presence of the other person. We don't need to be apprehensive about unpleasant surprises. We don't need to be afraid. There is need that later turns into desire, and the desire turns into determination. From need to desire, and then from desire to determination. It is better to breastfeed the baby than to bottle-feed them because, for the child, it is a miracle that their mother can survive their greed, their sucking her breasts. And this will have consequences in their thinking. When the mother feeds her baby from a bottle, she is protecting herself, she is not giving herself but something else. But when the child empties the mother's breast and it fills up again three hours later, that's a miracle. And yes, we need these miracles because they mean, for example, that we will not be afraid to ask for what we want. We know that the other person will survive our willpower. We don't need to fear for them.

Ronnie calls regression "neogenesis".[36] He also has the notion that our intellect, our mind that we don't know about, knows about us. And, of course, another very important idea of his – one that will stay with me for the rest of my life, I think – is that the patient is a person we accept, not an object we try to change.

I speak about Julian at Ronnie's seminar and, based on what I said, Ronnie decides that he no longer wants to be involved in his therapy. The only thing he was prepared to do, if necessary, is to work with the parents. We talk about the politics of therapy, about how we can't protect Julian from what is happening if we don't have enough power. We can't protect him from his parents. So, this isn't just therapy, it is politics, too. We do need to read Niccolò Machiavelli about the art of acquiring power and then holding onto that power, not losing it.[37] The therapist must know how to get enough power in their practice, in their life, to be able to do what they want and not do what they don't want. It is not power over others that we need, but power to prevent others from having power over us. Yes, this can be taught. This can be passed on.

Mike Yokum, Ronnie's student and one of our colleagues, tells us about a 50-year-old woman he is working with. The woman has an orgasm every time she sees a pipe sticking out of a wall, or when she hears several people stirring their cups of tea with a spoon in a café. She is hearing voices, and she has a sense of someone constantly watching her. She is always travelling. She can't stay in one place, she says she can understand the future, glimpse into people's souls and thoughts, and see things that are very far away. Ronnie suggests that Mike, first of all, study the facts: how old she is, whether she has siblings, where she was born, who her parents are – all the specifics. Then he can carry out specific observations like gestures, choreography, tone of voice, etc. And after all that, he may make conjectures. Something may have happened in the period before birth, before embedding, when communication channels are still open in every direction. Information comes from all directions for the blastula. Its biochemistry can sense every noise, every vibration. The nervous system only develops later on, and its function will be to filter out those things necessary for survival from all the cosmic music. But during this early phase, the womb and the mother's whole body, her hormones, are all "watching'" the blastula. This woman feels that she is being watched, like when she was a blastula. She is scared of real contact, and that is the reason for her constant movement. It's as if she is afraid of arriving. The blastula is constantly on the move. As long as it is in motion, the next step, embedding, has certainly not taken place. Maybe there is some trauma there, something bad that happened at that stage. It is a brave hypothesis, and it would be futile to try to prove it scientifically…

I was immediately attracted to the metaphor of perinatal theories as soon as I first heard them, although as a mathematician and physicist, I could never believe in this perspective. Today, I am certain that memory is a broader concept than its present scientific conceptualisation. I have had several discussions with Rupert Sheldrake (he holidays on Cortes Island, like me) about the existence of as yet undiscovered and unnamed biological fields; besides the magnetic field there are biological fields. Biologists don't really take him seriously, but he has proven empirically the existence of morphogenetic fields. He believes that every cell, including the zygote I had once been, has memory.

I decide to read everything by Winnicott.

I attend Heaton's group, too. He talks about how the therapist should get close to their patient, yet it is a problem if they get too close, while staying too distant also creates difficulties. One shouldn't be afraid of their own authority, says Heaton. There are therapists who are afraid to express what they know, what they are certain about. But one has to accept that the patient considers the therapist great. One shouldn't pretend this not to be the case. Every therapist should take his own authority seriously. They shouldn't feel bad about having power. They shouldn't feel guilty for asking for money for their work. If someone else pays on the patient's behalf, that is fine, but if, for example, the husband pays for the wife's therapy, that can create complications. This needs to be discussed, but it doesn't make work impossible, only more complicated.

Supervision with Ronnie. We talk about Anna, who wants to take medication so she can sleep. I told her that instead of taking sleeping pills, she should write down what she thinks or talk into her Dictaphone, so we can understand the situation. Ronnie snaps at me. I am cruel, he says. If she wants to take something, let her take it. Ronnie also hates it when he can't sleep. He asks for Novocaine at the dentist. He takes sleeping pills and antibiotics when he has an inflammation. It's no good not having medicine. Who do I think I am, forcing my prejudices on Anna? If Anna wants to go to hospital, let her go. I shouldn't stigmatise her because, if I do, I'll just become another male in her life who looks at her like she is a walking disaster, a person who can't make good decisions. I shouldn't expect anything from her. Supervision with Ronnie doubles as therapy. We talk about the origin of this rigidity in me, how I lost my flexibility. He deems it rigidness and heartlessness that, even for a moment, I disapproved of Anna wanting to take sleeping pills. Love and empathy demand that I should be her accomplice, that I shouldn't criticise her, and that I should understand her. I lived through terrible times, more horrifying than I would care to remember, and my survival strategy may have been becoming stoic, but I shouldn't demand the same from Anna. Anna may benefit from a sanatorium, nurses and lots of sleep. Just because I can't see myself in that situation, doesn't mean I should deprive Anna of it. Why do I make her life more difficult with my own personal ideological dilemma? This is not a question of ideology, but a question of love. I meet Anna later on, and to my relief she is well, she had a good sleep. I didn't create a big problem. I understand that by thinking in this way, there is a risk of considering Anna an idiot, and she will get the impression that she is incapable of making good decisions. And anyway, I am not the only smart man in the world looking after her. I don't necessarily know better than her what is good for her. It is complicated. One thinks one is being paid because one knows better what is good for the other person and to give advice. Ronnie thinks my advice to Anna was somewhat cruel, and I immediately sensed that he was right.

Winnicott talks about how someone who has really deep disassociations, someone who can't get in touch with their dreams, who has a huge chasm between their dreams and themself, would stay in touch with their dreams by compulsively projecting them into reality and acting them out. The reason for someone doing bizarre things may be their inability to dream. The closer they get to their dreams, the less they do outrageous things. If Hitler could have dreamt that he burnt the Jews, he wouldn't have had to do it in reality.

Ronnie and Judith Herman[38] agree about memories resurfacing when one is no longer afraid of them. The more fear is associated with memories, the less we can remember. Ronnie didn't think we had to remember everything to become cured. Years later, one of my patients, Janet – you can see this in a film – was trying to remember what her father did to her.[39] Ronnie looked at Janet with great love and said, "Listen, your future doesn't depend on what your father did. Imagine that he did all the horrendous things you can think of and start living the way you like, nevertheless!" He also told Janet not to be dogmatic. No need to remember until you can remember accurately.

This meeting today is typical. I have a cold, and we move onto practical things from the theoretical stuff. Ronnie explains to me how to rinse out my sinuses.

Recipe:
A cup of lukewarm water
1/4 teaspoon baking soda
1/4 teaspoon salt
Mix them well.
Gargle and irrigate the nose, morning and evening.

He is quite friendly now, friendlier than at other times. He tells me how fast time is passing for him. He is sympathetic towards me. He is trying to imagine my impressions after spending a few months here. He suspects that I consider people and situations life-threatening: either sink or swim. It would appear – he pats me on the shoulder – I am swimming.

I repress my own suffering. I turn away from my own anger and pain. Leon is unrestrained in flooding those around him with stuff I think should be kept inside. What is right? How should I experience suffering? Am I defective? "Good questions," says Ronnie. There are no answers. When Buddha speaks about life being suffering, that is a mistranslation. From birth to death, we live through so many losses, everything passes on, we have to take leave of everything, and that's life. Pain is inevitable. Buddha spoke against attachment. You don't even need to be attached to your own pain and suffering. Buddha really annoys Buddhists, as Christ annoys Christians. Unfortunately, we have this Buddha; unfortunately, we have this Christ, they say.

Francis's father, Julian Huxley, received several sets of electroshocks. It was his own choice. Sometimes they work, and they can be effective. Even nowadays, there are waiting lists for the machines, so many people want them. One can become addicted to them like heroin addiction. Julian was a young father. A nice, kind person. Everything was fine, but one day, he turned inward. For a full year, he just sat and thought. Then he got a series of ECTs and went back to normal.[40] That's it. And sometimes it works. Ronnie met 70-year-old people who had spent 50 years sitting in this type of deep contemplation, and it may be negligence leaving someone in that state. Maybe if one gets a set of ECTs at 20, one can go on to live a good life. "I would never allow them to do that to me," says Ronnie, "but if that's what one of my patients wants, then why not? It's perfectly fine."

I am reading Erik Erikson's *Insight and Responsibility*.[41] He says we can't just study the human mind. One has to be with one's patient with one's full heart and soul, like a partner. You can't be an outside observer. You can only see a relationship from inside, otherwise you won't notice the things in others that you have never noticed in yourself.

For a long time, I wanted to understand myself, to know myself, and I thought I could get to know the other person too, but this is just misleading scientific posing. One has to be careful because it is easy to colonise the other person when one tries to fit them into what one already knows. But the categories of the other person may be inconceivably and infinitely different from my own. I don't have to get to know them, I don't have to analyse them in detail, I just have to love them, accept them and take delight in them. Acceptance doesn't depend on understanding.

Francis tells us about the Bushman people. He used to live among them, for a long time. The guys walk around with a hard-on. All the men walk around with erections, as if they were ashamed of having a soft cock. They drink a thick black beverage, which is supposed to be life-giving. Francis doesn't know what it is made of. He thinks it is some homeopathic stuff to deal with shame. "There are lots of medicines," he says, "that work by slightly altering the experience, the consciousness." He is not sure whether it is the chemical that works. Sometimes one just needs the experience to change and then one can use it for whatever is necessary, one can heal oneself. The medicine is just there to indicate that change is possible. If someone tells me, "Hey, you have black spots on your face!" I can reply, "Isn't it brilliant?" You can be proud of anything that you can be ashamed of. You can live free from shame, not being ashamed of even black spots on your face. Psychotherapy can also be used to humiliate oneself, but equally for elevating oneself, too. The only psychotherapy techniques Francis doesn't like are the ones without love, like Arica. Laura, Aldous's wife, says that "you are the goal". The goal is that whoever is with you should focus on loving you. Krishnamurti and Aldous unanimously told Francis during a discussion that if you think there is a problem, then the solution is letting go of the idea of the problem. So, you don't have to solve it, it is enough to let go. Krishnamurti thinks that all techniques are from the devil. He says he never did anything good on purpose. When he does something good, it's always by accident. Using a technique is wilful. One wilfully wants to do good. The therapist tells the patient that we will make a birth tunnel for you, and you have to go through it. Then the spirit of the exercise is that it will benefit the patient. The patient is somewhat hypnotised by the knowledge that the therapist will be pleased if the exercise benefits them. But if it happens to occur to me, how much fun it would be to play a game with a birth tunnel, I feel like doing it, you feel like doing it, so let's see what will happen, well then, that's a game, not a technique. Playing with techniques is fine. A game is a game because there is no consequence. This is my impression here at the Philadelphia Association, at the seminars and workshops, that everything is playful. In one of the groups, Ronnie says that if anyone wants, they can wrestle with him, just because one can also play with the body, and wrestling is an experience. One doesn't know where it will lead to. He once kicked Leon so hard, he couldn't walk for weeks.

Winnicott says that if he had to select a colleague as a therapist, or for a psychoanalysis training, he would prefer to choose someone who has the disposition or talent for this work, rather than someone who has suffered a lot and got better through therapy.[42] I ponder this. This is the exact opposite of what Ronnie says about shamans. He doesn't think of psychosis as an illness, but as the road to enlightenment. In Greek, *metanoia* is when one's heart and mind transform.[43] That is enlightenment, but the road from normal to metanoia goes through paranoia. It has to do with South American shamans and Alcoholics Anonymous where the helper, shaman or sponsor must be someone who has "come through" the illness or affliction. With AA, part of the healing is the awareness that, sooner or later, one must heal others. If one avoids that, one will relapse. Still, Winnicott would choose someone with a talent over someone who needs to be cured first. One who is cured in therapy will certainly have more faith in the effectiveness of therapy because it worked for them. Winnicott says we should allow for, or admit, that it is always better that someone has never suffered than being cured of one's suffering.

Trauma also has a good aspect, but it is still better not to suffer traumas. Those who don't have to suffer are fortunate. He would want someone with a good family, good education, good friends, good spouse and good life as his therapist. Ronnie tells me that we shouldn't think that the world is just full of suffering people, just because we spend most of our time with the afflicted. There are some fortunate people who have no idea what we are talking about. They have no need for us. They live their lives energetically and happily, with no dilly-dally. Rather than being envious of them, we should be happy they exist.

I have seen, several times, that marriage and family become one's old family, and sex and romance is found elsewhere. According to Ronnie, this is a European tradition, and I should read Denis de Rougemont's book, *Love in the Western World*, about French families and love.

In Erikson's book, I read about how it is not sufficient for the patient's symptoms to disappear for us to pronounce them cured. They are only cured when they have the energy and concentration for projects that are important to them: work, family, friendships and the world. Settling in the world is the standard for being well enough, not the absence of symptoms. Similarly, according to Freud, therapy has ended when the patient becomes so busy that they forget about the session, when their own affairs become more important than therapy.

Party at Ronnie's tonight. His mood is weird. When we arrive, he says he is despairing, and he expects us boys and girls to cheer him up. He seems to have lost his way. He has to redeem the cosmos. He is brooding over why the cosmos needs him, and why he needs the cosmos. He is unsure about whether he can believe what he says. The notions and insights of prenatal and perinatal psychology appear to be valid, but it is just as plausible that we are projecting things into early life, and none of this is actually true. But even if it is true, what does it have to do with love and compassion? If love and compassion are important, who the hell cares about prenatal and perinatal psychology? He categorically states that things that are not connected to love and compassion have to be endured, and then left behind as soon as possible. Yet a little while later, he talks about how the manner of one's birth – how the baby emerges, head first or feet first – shapes one's future character. He is positive that those who are lifted from the mother's abdomen by caesarean section, without undergoing labour, live their lives differently from those who passed through the birth canal. I can sense that Leon and Ronnie are close. They support each other. They sing. I am listening to them sing "Nobody knows the trouble I've seen", and I weep.[44] Then they sing Christmas songs and old hits from the 1920s. Jutta, Ronnie's wife, retires early, then she reappears occasionally, to tell us we are too loud. They start reading the Bible. Ronnie has ideas, for example, that the members of the Philadelphia Association should record their own readings of the whole Bible. Ronnie says there are certain chapters in the Bible that make him cry. He tears up as soon as he reads them. He doesn't need to feel or think anything, the tears just start flowing. These teardrops are like the drops of blood coming from the severed umbilical cord, when we feel cut off from something. We talk about Oedipus, who cries drops of blood.

They read *Four Quartets* by T.S. Eliot, including the opening poem, "Burnt Norton". Ronnie reads wonderfully. The reading continues. Leon reads from Genesis, and David Goldblatt from the Book of Psalms. I ask Ronnie what makes him so dejected, what is so hopeless. "I, myself," he says. "Do you think you are not needed?" I carry on, quizzing him. "No, no, Jutta thinks that." I meant cosmically, I tell him, and he replies that that question is not whether the cosmos needs him but whether he needs the cosmos, this whole thing.

This subject, namely what was his purpose in this world, often came up with Laing, up until the end of his life, especially when he was drunk. With tears in his eyes, he would say that he was expected on the other side, that there was a string quartet there waiting for a pianist. They want to play with him, and he would much rather be there than here. Once, there was a party in Vancouver, Ram Dass[45] was there too, and I was talking with Ronnie in the kitchen. He was smoking. Ram Dass came in all white and bright. "Ronnie, you smoke?" he asked. Ronnie looked at him derisively, "If I didn't have the taste and fragrance of cigarettes, I wouldn't even be on this earth any more. This is the only thing keeping me here because the company, you for example, is not worth staying for, even for one minute." His depression stemmed from deep hopelessness. Like the Spanish *noche oscura*, the title of one of Saint John's poems, "The Dark Night", about the dark night of the soul, Ronnie felt disconnected, cut off from God, humans, spirit, love, certainty, faith and hope. He was praying for it all to end, he was searching for signs, but nothing happened. Once I asked him why he didn't kill himself. He said he considered suicide insolent and cheeky, and he didn't want to be insolent. The universe had created him, so he didn't want to be ungrateful, but he also didn't want to prolong his life, just like Rilke.[46] He thought that one's life was one's own experience, and one's death was also one's own experience, dying being a part of life. One has to experience their own death. They shouldn't try to run away from it. Rilke suffered from very painful anaemia, but he didn't see a doctor, and he died like an animal. Ronnie didn't see a doctor either. He was bleeding, but he didn't want to know why. He was hoping he would die sooner rather than later. When, after he died, I was reading his diary notes, I realised that during his last three years, he suffered from a lot of pain, but every day he had a few hours when he could write, and he felt very grateful for that. He died while playing tennis with Robert Firestone.[47] Whenever Ronnie was feeling a bit better, he used to help Firestone write his book on a yacht. He collapsed during a game, and they rushed to him, telling him that the doctor was on his way. He started swearing – fuck off, who the hell needs a doctor, I am a doctor too, I don't need a doctor – and he died. Did he need the cosmos? What was good for him? What did he get from the cosmos? Towards the end, he was definitely bored. He either scared people off or found them boring, and he was left increasingly on his own. After losing Jutta, his wife, he was mostly on his own. Jutta felt he didn't need her. She preferred to be the beloved in a relationship rather than the lover. When Ronnie first met her, he showered her with love, and she was the centre of the universe. But later on, he didn't pay enough attention to her because of his work. She found herself a lover at an international conference and they used to meet in secret.

When Ronnie found out, he was heartbroken, especially because Jutta lied to him. That's when he started writing *The Lies of Love*. The book is still unpublished. I have the manuscript. It is in fragments, and it isn't edited. He wrote parts of it here in Vancouver, and one of my patients did the typing for him. Marguerite, his last girlfriend, the mother of his tenth child, wants to get it published because she says Ronnie gave her this book.

There are many abandoned houses in London where homeless people can squat. They don't pay for anything, and if they can, they use the gas and electricity until they get thrown out. Ronnie lived in one of these houses and Marguerite, his secretary, lived there with him because she felt sorry for him. They had a child together when Ronnie was 60. He died at 62. Charles is his last son. Another of his sons, Adrian, who is the executor of Ronnie's legacy, won't allow the book to be published. He is a stuck-up middle-class Scotsman who calls Marguerite's son a bastard, and calls his father a bastard, too, because he begot a son outside of wedlock. The nerve! Marguerite wrote to me that we should publish it, together with commentaries, but Adrian calls me a bastard, too, because when I got married to my wife, Meredith, we already had Marcel and Meredith was pregnant with Soma. This is the way it is in Scotland, Adrian says, and Ronnie was Scottish. I think the book is a little feeble. There isn't enough kick to it, and we never find out why the cosmos needed Ronnie. Anyway, Marguerite and I are thinking about our options.

At 1 a.m., I get a taxi home. At eight in the morning, I am rushing back to therapy. It seems like I have caught Ronnie's depression, I feel awful. Just as I arrive, Ronnie pulls up in a Mini with a big red L plate: learner driver. Jutta is waiting for him at the door. She is furious with him for being late. She needs to go somewhere. We go in, but I don't feel I have anything to say. I sit there in silence. Maybe I've dreamt something, and that's why I don't feel like doing anything. Ronnie asks me whether I often feel like this, and does this remind

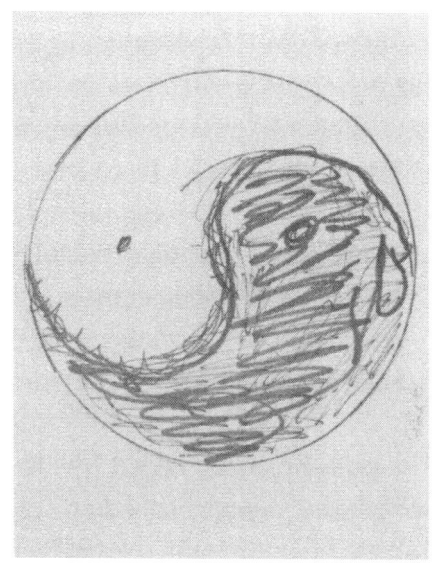

me of anything. As it happens, when someone hurts me, for example, when my wife is upset and angry, I always fall asleep. Ronnie asks me whether he upset me the night before because, as usual, he doesn't remember anything. No, he didn't upset me, I tell him, but I had a thought about his depression. I make a drawing for him. People living on the middle line between the white and the black have a harder time than those in the middle of the white or black bits.

On the border, in the not-this and not-that existence, one is extremely creative, but one doesn't know where one belongs. Ronnie definitely doesn't belong to any trend, ideology or school of thought. I think his depression stems from this. This is why he is unsure of whether the cosmos needs him. I try to comfort him by telling him that, if with nothing else, he is definitely helping the universe by making so many babies. Jutta is expecting Ronnie's eighth child. I ask him whether it is possible that his depression is due to Jutta being pregnant. No, he says. I tell him how a breeze caressed my face as I was walking here, as if the fragrance of a long-gone rose garden touched me, a memory from when I was 14, and I felt this huge emotion welling up in me, I became tearful. A painful nostalgia for something that's lost forever. I admit that I cried yesterday too, when they were singing. Even he couldn't understand my experience, and it made me feel so lonely. Nobody understands it. Ronnie looks at me, and asks whether I often allowed myself to have these feelings. No, I say. And that's it.

> At that time, I didn't manage to articulate it, but now I know that I felt excluded that night when Ronnie just played the piano, and I only saw his back all night. Many people sang together, but I don't remember the words of the songs.

I am reading Erikson, who says that reliable motherhood needs a reliable cosmos, and women's religiousness or faith is different from men's.[48] Women's faith is much less dependent on logic, while male logic has no compunction about any kind of action. It is the responsibility of women to give hope and faith to new people, and logic doesn't exonerate them from this duty. It is terrifying to contemplate, but if a generation of mothers can't trust and hope, that would be the end of humanity. Hope is completely illogical, but we perish without hope.

Hugh Crawford talks about Theodor Schwenk's book, *Sensitive Chaos*. It is about water and how water is alive. It can take on various shapes, and it is proven scientifically that it remembers and has a tendency to create spheres. You can meditate on anything. Anything may be an object of meditation. One can contemplate the phenomenology of things. There is a French writer, Gaston Bachelard, who writes brilliant books on the phenomenology of fire and water.[49] When he meditates on water, he can

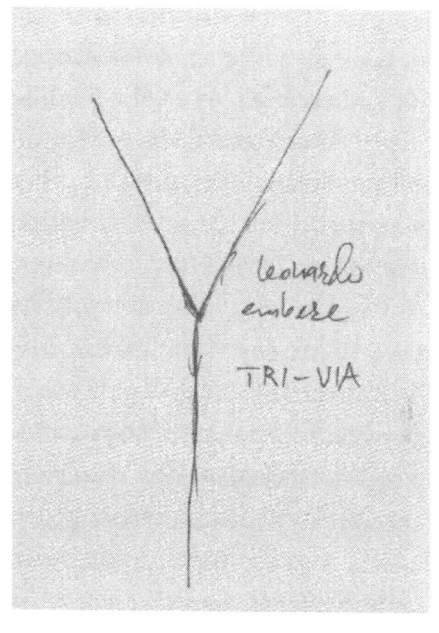

sense infinity and feel that this mystery has no beginning and no end. We use it, it surrounds us, and it is a miracle we don't even notice. We know nothing about it. It is very important for us to be inquisitive and to search for the origin of things. Whatever has life gives birth. We live in time. We are all like a little whirlpool or wave: we begin in the water, we change and we disappear. Each of us is an event. We don't exist in time, but we are events of time. Time creates us, and we are time. We know there is a past, but we can't go there. There is a future, but we can't go there, either.

We are constantly at a fork in the road, where the road divides into two. No matter where we came from, we constantly must choose. This is the "Y," the *tri via*, which means "three roads", where one road splits into two. If I stop at this point, don't make a decision, don't choose, and I don't move in either direction, then my life becomes trivial.

Therapy is not psychology. I am born into this world, and no one knows what my purpose is. There is no pattern, no plan, and no blueprint. But through me, through my words, something is definitely presented and expressed in the world. Words are dangerous, like dynamite, like fire, but they shouldn't be avoided. Some people know the power of words, and that's the reason they don't talk. They are afraid of this power.

Where do babies come from? This is a big question. We have to keep asking this question. We were all conceived and born, we are all fruits of a madness that continually bears fruit, and we are all ambrosia or wafer in the mouths of gods.

The etymology of "psychology" is *psyche*, or "soul" and *-logy* or "study of". In "psychiatry", the "-iatry" comes from *iatreia*, which means care and healing, so "psychiatry" means healing of the soul.

The Ten Commandments are not commandments, and they are especially not a series of prohibitions. They are a phenomenological description of what will happen when one reaches the stage of existence where God is. At that stage, one will not do the things that are prohibited in the Ten Commandments. It is very important that we don't grow up obeying. This is crucial. The best way for a two-year-old to become a five-year-old is to be loved. Nobody will become a five-year-old quicker if they have to act as if they were five, even though they are just two. People who are forced to obey become patients in my practice.

It is a grave mistake to show a child an adult and expect them to behave like that adult. That makes the child lose their own existence. This is the first step in thinking. Lacan writes about the mirror stage that we all go through. A baby's subjective experience, until the age of 10 or 12 months, is that when they are sucking the breast, they are a big mouth. The rest of their body is limp, they are not in their feet, so they are not one with their whole body. You can see it in their eyes that when they are having a poop, they are where the pooping happens. They disappear from their eyes, and they are not present. When they see themselves in the mirror and realise that what they see is themselves, and they are one whole thing, that's when the ideal ego starts. And we torment ourselves with this ideal ego. According to Lacan, the I is always worse than the ideal. Thinking that the Ten Commandments is an ideal that we should compare ourselves to is a misinterpretation of the Ten Commandments. Due to this misunderstanding, we are continually torturing ourselves. Every time Winnicott spoke to mothers, he made it clear that it was more important for them to be themselves than to be "Winnicottian mothers". Ronnie is right, the only things that are actually important are compassion and love. I have several patients who are ruthless with themselves. One of them wanted to be a screenwriter as a young man. He wanted to work with the world's best directors, like Wim Wenders and Ingmar Bergman. Now, he looks at his successful colleagues as Antonio Salieri looked at Wolfgang Amadeus Mozart in Peter Shaffer's play, *Amadeus*. Salieri blasphemes God. He knows what is good, he enjoys Mozart's music, but he cannot compose anything like that. Why does God give one the talent to see what is good without also providing him with the talent to be able to do it? When this happens, one either wants to destroy oneself or the ideal. The only thing I can do with my patient is to try to convince him that it is better to love himself, and that he shouldn't destroy himself with competition and comparisons. But he can't imagine life without being special, outstanding, beyond compare. His agony is truly heart-rending.

I start reading Freud's book *Totem and Taboo*. I really like the ideas that madness is a caricature of art, compulsive neurosis is a parody of religion and paranoid delusions and hallucinations satirise philosophy. Another interesting notion is that turning away from reality is the same as turning away from human society. Ronnie also read this very attentively, and it confirmed his belief that madness is probably motivated by being torn, by being in a company one doesn't want to be in as a child. Freud's patient, Little Hans, was terrified of everything hairy. If a woman appeared in a fur coat, he would run away in terror. Freud and the child's father manage to find out that when Hans was little, he was once lying in his pram, and a big dog barked into his face. That fear later became associated with everything hairy, and he became terrified of everything hairy. A person who goes mad becomes fearful of everyone and doesn't say, well, my mother hurt me, or my father hurt me, but rather that people are all like that. Therapy is often like teaching a Little Hans that he only has to be afraid of certain dogs and not of everything hairy. The only way for him to accept this is by stepping over his fears, by someone he trusts taking him to a fur coat and laying him down there. Although he feels aversion, two minutes later, he can play with the fur. Sometimes, the therapist is the first person in someone's life who doesn't hurt them. It is crucial for the therapist to communicate to the patient that they are not going to hurt them, to communicate harmlessness non-verbally, through their being. I am hairy, but I don't bark. Then the patient can learn to stop generalising.

Ronnie seems tired. He is listening with his eyes closed, or he may be sleeping. I don't say anything. I don't talk. Whenever someone asks him not to close his eyes when they are talking to him, he tells them to fuck off. He can be perfectly attentive, even with his eyes closed. No one can demand anything from him. I speak about three things. One is that I am in deep shit in terms of money. I've run out of what I've brought with me, and I don't make enough. Still, I ask him to have three sessions a week, not just two. I tell him four dream fragments. He apologises for not speaking a lot. He is sorry I happened to come to London in the middle of a global economic recession, and he doesn't have many patients either. His Mondays are free. He will think about having three sessions a week. He doesn't say a word about the dreams, only I mention them.

The greengrocer where I usually do my shopping is an old Pakistani man, and he calls me professor. I go shopping with Soma, holding her hand. I go to the counter with my basket to pay. It is a pound and a penny. I am rummaging in my left pocket, fish out a penny, and give it to the old guy. Then I get a pound out of my right pocket to give to him, but he gently pushes my hand away and doesn't accept the money. He is satisfied with the penny. All my depression evaporates. This is a sign that money will come. If even this little old Pakistani man is giving me money, then there is no problem.

We are drinking wine at Francis's seminar. His definition of wine is "correctly managed corruption". Corruption is the rotting. The lovely grapes start rotting, but if the rotting is taken care of properly, the grapes become good wine. As an anthropologist, he says sometimes it is difficult to sink from the light of mythology into the darkness of logic, causes and effects. He thinks laughter is the cure against taboos. He studied the Kwakiutl indigenous peoples, the "capitalists" of North America.[50] They were capitalists because property and wealth were important to them. In ancient times, people of this culture were not intoxicated by wine but by human flesh. One can get drunk on horror. In life, black is entwined with white and the external is entwined with the internal. This twisting can only be understood if one is drunk, and one really needs to laugh. Laughing is the greatest understanding. There is a difficult alternative to laughing, throwing up, which is very deep laughter. Vomiting is part of the ayahuasca ritual. The twisting snake is sex and intelligence, and we can give it a heart by making it drunk. The Brothers Grimm fairy tale of the boy who wants to learn to shiver, "The Story of the Youth Who Went Forth to Learn What Fear Was", is about this. Because we have to accept what's there: if there is fear, we have to shiver; if something is funny, we have to laugh. Everything that presents itself will also go away, so no need to be scared of anything, whatever is there is there. I give myself over to whatever is there. "Open

your tender underbelly to the sword of unwanted experience!"
as E.G. Howe says.[51]

Mina talks about how Ronnie selects his patients. He doesn't
work with just anyone. The person must possess intuitive intelligence, be good at expressing themselves, and have good verbal
skills for Ronnie to enjoy their company, and he must notice
a real desire for honesty. It is important to Ronnie that he can
imagine his patient emerging as a person who doesn't hurt others, a person who is able to love. If, somehow, he can't see this
possibility, he won't work with the person.

This is Tit-mouth. I draw
it for Ronnie, and he likes
it. This creature runs
around on chicken legs.
If it approaches you with
its breast at the front, you
can't see its mouth, and if
it comes towards you with
its mouth at the front, you
can't see its breast. It is a
simple diagram, facilitating a deep understanding
of the dynamics of rela-
tionships. When two Tit-
mouths meet, one of them
has its breast at the front
because it is ashamed of

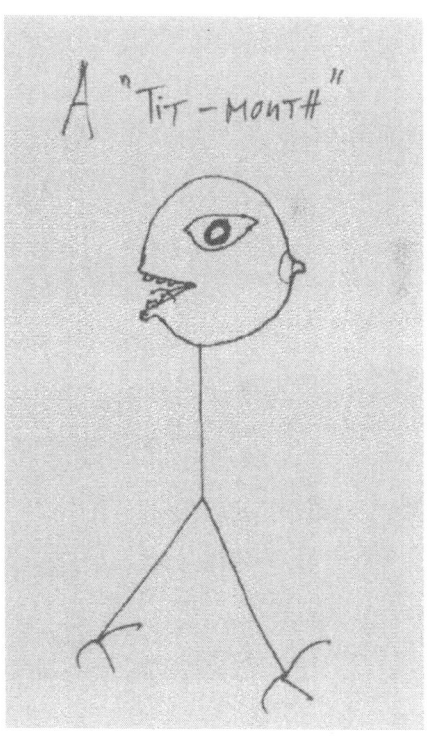

its mouth, and then the other thinks that this one doesn't have a mouth. And this other one, this has its mouth at the front and it hides its breast. Every combination is possible. When both Titmouths rotate, that's healing. They are going towards each other, and they both know that the other has a mouth and a breast too. So, neither of them has to be ashamed of anything. No need to be afraid that if one of them is too greedy or it doesn't have enough milk to give, the other will desert it. Thus, we are all Titmouths; we all have a mouth and a breast too, and we needn't hide anything.

The serpent, Ouroboros, is the symbol of will. If the serpent is willpower, then our most important task is to be resolute in not wanting anything. This can be the only true goal of willpower: to want not to want. Marion Milner points out often that the

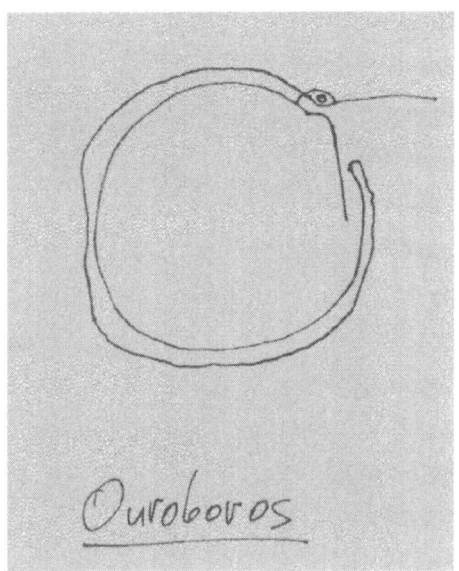

Ouroboros

only proper function of the will is to will not to will.[52] The Ouroboros serpent eating its own tail is a symbol of this. We short-circuit our wanting. If we already want, we give it its own tail to eat, then it will leave us alone. All anxiety originates from wanting, from not accepting what is, or from wanting something we can't will. Anxiety is a will-disorder. This becomes terribly disturbing. I want to fall asleep when I am not sleepy, I want to remember something or I want someone to like me: these are not things you can will. If it happens anyway, the best thing to do is feed my will to itself. I don't want to want to sleep. It's not my business. Whether someone likes me or not is not my business. If the other person knew or noticed that I am constantly working on trying to make them like me, they would feel attacked, or at least put off.

This image is a good start to get us contemplating the Kundalini metaphor. The Kundalini is sleeping, it is biting its own tail in its sleep, and it's down in the first chakra. It is preoccupied with itself and doesn't give me any energy. At least, that's the case when only survival matters. Even for sexual interests to awaken, Kundalini needs to let go of its tail and climb up to the next chakra, the genitals.

If life is like hanging on to a sheer vertical cliff face with bleeding nails, and there is a constant danger of falling, one doesn't have much energy for anything else. But if one manages to work one's way up to the top of the cliff, where one can lie down on a horizontal surface and feel safe, then sexual energy

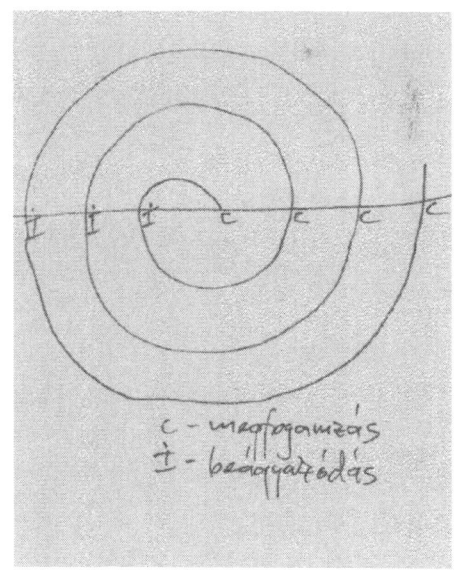

can start pulsating. One can allow oneself to smile at someone because one can do one's own thing without a constant fear of plunging to one's death. Well, this is Ouroboros or Kundalini.

Life is a snail. Let's start with the first "C" in the middle, for conception. The father's sperm meets the mother's ovum, and the next stage is "I", or implantation. Every "I" turns into a "C", and every "C" turns into an "I", until we die. Something new starts. This new thing has to be settled into the world. This is an endless series...

When Lili, the daughter of Réka and Attila (a Hungarian couple close to the Feldmár Institute) was conceived and began to grow inside her mother, that was something new. That being had never been inside Réka before. Lili became implanted in Réka's womb, but then she had to leave it, as one has to leave all implantations. Lili appeared, and then she had to be implanted in the world of her father and mother. Then another spark came, and she had to leave that world to be implanted in the nursery. I, for example, had to burst my way out of Hungary and become implanted in Canada. Each exit is an entry, and each entry is an exit. This never ends. Stanislav Grof and E.E. Cummings both write about humanity being the species that isn't born just once.

This triangle illustrates the mechanism of every rebirth. This is the engine, the holy trinity, of Hinduism. Brahma, the creator, constantly creates anew, Vishnu protects whatever is born, but Shiva, the destroyer, doesn't like it. Because he is bored with what's there, there is nothing there after all, so he destroys everything he can. He annihilates situations, structures, and customs. This, in turn, allows Brahma to create anew from the ruins, and Vishnu rushes to protect it. This goes on forever. A good Hindu will pray in the temples of all three deities and offer gifts to all of them.

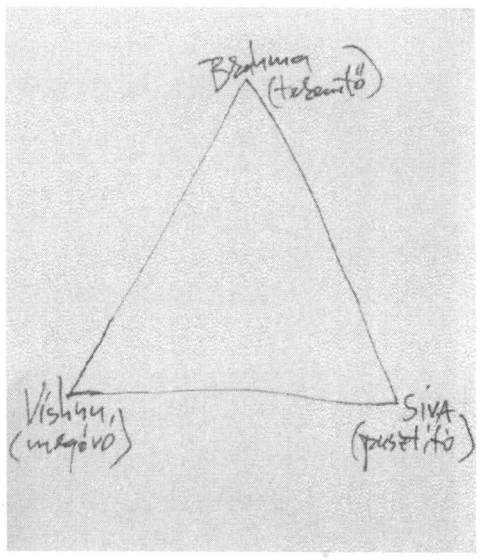

But there are many of us who are afraid of one aspect or another. But if we avoid one of them, we are in trouble. The purpose of this is an infinite game: just keep it going.

In my work with Laing, the possibility emerged of leaving everything behind in Vancouver and moving to London for good. Ruptures are always started by Brahma or Shiva. When I was moaning about how difficult it was to make money, I was begging Vishnu to protect me from having to go back early. Then one day, I decided to go back. One of the reasons was Marcel turning five, and if he had started school in London in September 1975, then a couple of years later, I would have had to pluck him out of his circle of friends when we moved back to Vancouver. I didn't think we would stay in London for eight years, and I thought it would be better to go somewhere where we could stay for at least eight years. I can coexist with

Shiva, but he needs Vishnu. The other reason was that I could see that, on that stage, I would only ever be a prince, I could never become king. That was Ronnie's kingdom. I didn't like the rivalry of the other princes, and I didn't want to take part in it. I thought, in Vancouver, I could become the king. I felt a deep sense of sadness because it was nice living in Ronnie's kingdom, but I had to leave him to be able to create and build my own kingdom. My son followed the same path: as soon as he could become independent, he immediately moved to Seattle and then to L.A. Here in Vancouver, people used to say, "There is Marcel, Andrew Feldmár's son." But now, when I go to Los Angeles, I am "Marcel Feldmar's father". He is the king there, and that is the way it should be. If one's father is very strong, it is difficult to grow up to become a king in the father's kingdom, and Marcel, like the prince of fairy tales, found his own kingdom. I often invited Ronnie to my own kingdom, but that was different, we worked together. Staying with him for that one year was enough for me. That was the reason for my fervent note-taking – it was my way of packing. I knew I would have everything I needed. I would just have to unpack it from my notes. This way, I didn't have to stay longer. Freud worked long days, and he never took notes. It was never like how they depict him in the pictures. But at the end of the day, he sat down and wrote everything he remembered. He trusted his memory, and he trusted that he would remember everything that was really important. He knew he only had to write down what he remembered because only that was important. I did the same thing. I learned from Ronnie, who also didn't write much, but every morning and evening, he noted down whatever was important to him. This is how I wrote the notes that gave birth to this book, to *Credo*. I have several patients who record each session on their phones. I don't tell them not to do it, but I have a good laugh to myself. It is as if they are scared to become absorbed in the present, and they only open up to a discussion when they are safely on their own. They are scared of arguing with me, so they pluck up their courage when I am not there any longer. They say that when I'm not present, and they are having imaginary conversations with me, I say much better things than in real life, when present.

At his seminar, Ronnie speaks about the organism being in a particular environment from the moment it comes into existence. He believes that therapy is a practice of modifying the environment without hurting the organism. We encourage our patients with examples, and we make it clear that, from the age of 16, we are all responsible for our own environment. This, of course, is true not just for our physical environment.

I think that should be ingrained in the brains of anyone who wants to work with people. When I am invited to see a family in which the teenage son is breaking and destroying everything, scaring his mom and dad, and whose parents call for me to tame the boy, I go as a midwife to help the boy be born, and leave his family with the least possible amount of pain. Then he can find an environment where he doesn't become angry and he doesn't have to threaten anyone. I am surprised this is not obvious, and that there are therapists who try to bully the teenager into behaving nicely.

A woman gives birth to her third child and then sinks into a deep depression, which is called "postpartum depression" by the psychiatric profession, and which is treated accordingly. The poor, sick mother is put on medication. But the real problem is that her husband carried on with life as if nothing had happened, she didn't get any extra support when the new baby came, and she realised that instead of being on the brink of freedom, after two kids, she was in for another 3–4 years of prison to look forward to. So, I work with the husband and the wife, and we look into whether the husband could be more understanding and helpful.

Sometimes I am attacked and I get thrown out. I am told I am incompetent because I am not making a diagnosis, and I don't agree that the problem is with the woman. They take the woman to the doctor and she is put on medication. Then they cheerfully tell me that everything is fine. The foundation is always to find the site of the trouble: is it within a person or is it between people? The therapist's room is a different environment from the one the patient is escaping from. In the secure environment I can provide, the patient is able to sink into their traumas and wounds that they got outside. These, cannot be resolved logically, in their head. But a safe environment will alleviate their fears. According to Laing, the patient's every cell must sense that there is no need to be afraid here, and then they can develop hope that an outside environment exists where they would not be abused. Once they have this knowledge deep down, they can create such environments for themself.

Ronnie says that fear's headquarters is in the bone marrow; that's where terror starts. Blood cells are produced here, and blood transports fear to every cell, including the brain, of course. Being healed or curing someone must reach the cytoplasm. In other words, when someone is hurt, an alarm bell goes off, and with the help of the therapist the patient has to find this alarm bell. Knowing that the danger has passed, they can switch it off. It is crucial, therefore, that the therapist is there without any of their sounds and moves, signalling danger.

Everything we really enjoy doing can make us money. How? Ronnie loves being with his children, and the only way he can make money from it is by writing a book on the time they spend together. If one's energy processes are not clogged up, one can adjust practically all one's enjoyable activities to make some money from them. Money is not the goal, it's just the extra. I oscillate between an intense passivity and making enthusiastic efforts. When I am passive, I am just waiting for the world to give me what I want. My mother said I was waiting for the pie in the sky. Then I suddenly shift from this extreme passivity into working hard and catching hold of every opportunity. Ronnie tells me that when he moved to London from Scotland, he lived far from the city centre. He had to work, and he already had four children. He used to commute two and a half hours, twice a day, so he used his time on the train to learn German. He offers practical help, so I can make money: I could have a group in his house or in Crawford's house. He trusts me. One of his patients has a computer business and Ronnie asks him if he could make use of me. I contemplate my passivity. Somehow, I yearn for not having to grow up, I give the world a chance to take care of me, and I hanker after a good mother. My mother used to make fun of me for wanting a good mother. I am an idiot waiting for the pie in the sky. I wanted her to take care of me and provide me with whatever I needed, but instead she expected me to provide her with what she needed. I am afraid to ask, and that doesn't make things easier, but there is also this thing of having to remain invisible. If I ask, I become visible. Ronnie called my diffidence "reverse arrogance". He challenged me to ask for what was there for the asking.

> Sheldon Kopp's message to beginner therapists is that only two things are important: one is to make yourself visible, because if you are hiding, no one will know that you exist; and the other is to work well, do your work to a high standard, and stay in the same place for a long time, so people can depend on you. These two pieces of advice really worked for me, and if a young therapist asks me for advice, I say the same.

Ronnie invites Heinz Cassirer for a discussion. Only seven of us are allowed to be present as an audience. They talk about the lineage and history of thoughts. They go back to Greek and Hebrew roots. They both possess an incredible depth and wealth of knowledge. The best thing would be for me to go home right now and just read for ten years to even get an idea of what they are talking about. It is a long discussion, but there is no emotion whatsoever. They read out quotes and ideas and debate them. It is exciting beyond belief. I would have to spend half of my life in libraries to be able to take part in a discussion like this.

The next day, I admit to Ronnie how ignorant I feel. He tells me it isn't psychotherapy that will deal with the problem. He writes out a list of 12 books to read and hands me the paper like a prescription.[53] If I read these, I'll know the most important things about the history of European thought, and I will be able to understand the connections.

I have read them all very carefully, several times. The picture below shows my scribbles next to Ronnie's writing. I noted down which London bookshop would have a particular book. These texts are liberating. After reading them, I felt I could breathe more easily and think more skilfully and enthusiastically. These texts are encouraging, and they speak to the heart.

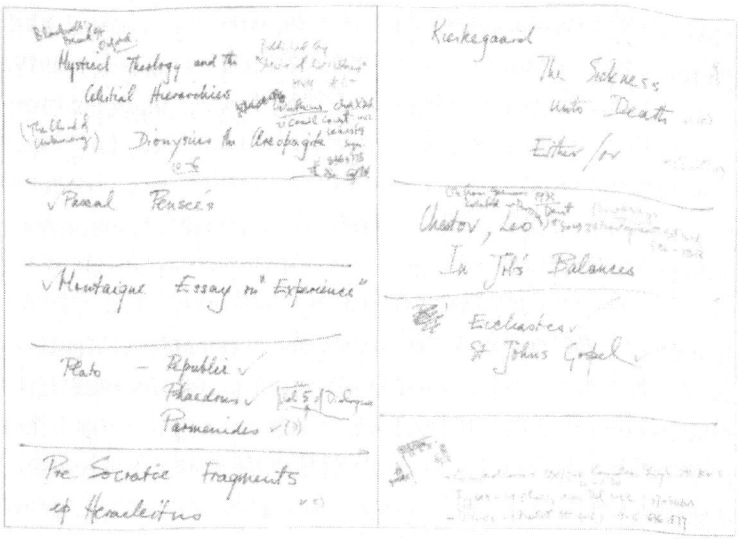

Cassirer speaks about how the circumcision of Jews is the sign or token of their covenant with God. He wasn't circumcised until the age of 71. He was translating the Bible at the time. He had the ritual done, and then he felt better. Until it took place, he didn't feel part of the Jewish community. Well, neither do I, I thought, but I don't think for me that's a big problem.

Ronnie reads the last two chapters of the Ecclesiastes, 11 and 12. Heinz tells us that between the ages of 31 and 51, he cut all connections with his mother. Well, it seems like he has issues with his mother too. He looks at me, and he says he can't see my face. Maybe it's because of the hair and beard, but there might be another reason. I feel ashamed, but it is interesting that he is looking for my face.

Ronnie thinks I would really enjoy Heinz's intellectual judo, and it's possible I would be just as vicious with him as Ronnie, if I didn't feel guilty for not having done my homework. Heinz accuses Ronnie of wasting his time on idiots. I don't want to be an idiot that Ronnie wastes his time on. Ronnie says he disagrees with Heinz, who wants him to spend all his time writing because that was more important than time spent with patients and students. Ronnie doesn't agree. He is sorry that he has to protect his associates when he invites Heinz. The last time Heinz visited, he hurt an American psychologist lady so deeply, she burst into tears. Ronnie is sorry that people don't stand up for themselves. They don't put their foot down when they come across challenges like the ones Heinz represents. Heinz is completely serious, but he says everything that occurs to him and usually everything that occurs to him is correct. But not always! When he met Leon, within five minutes, he figured him out and said everything about him that took Ronnie five years to discover. He said Leon was spiritually deaf. It's just as well I have a beard, and my face is invisible.

I talk with Ronnie about how I grew up with girls, while he only knew boys until the age of 17. His experiences were very different from mine. At the age of 11, he married a girl in the gang he belonged to, and the ceremony and everything gave him a very important emotional experience, but girls still remained strangers.

A naked man approached me, my bed, in a dream. Ronnie's interpretation is that the spirit of the Philadelphia Association is very masculine, and because I grew up with girls, I find this a problem. Penetration is very important in every encounter, not just in sexual ones. How we get on with each other depends on who penetrates whom; who receives and who gives.

I go to the shelter at Portland Road. I find a Bible, and I have a look at what he read from the Book of Ecclesiastes.

11.1. Cast thy bread upon the waters: for thou shalt find it after many days. 2. Give a portion to seven, and also to eight; for thou knowest not what evil shall be upon the earth. 3. If the clouds be full of rain, they empty themselves upon the earth: and if the tree fall toward the south, or toward the north, in the place where the tree falleth, there it shall be. 4. He that observeth the wind shall not sow; and he that regardeth the clouds shall not reap. 5. As thou knowest not what is the way of the spirit, nor how the bones do grow in the womb of her that is with child: even so thou knowest not the works of God who maketh all.

6. In the morning sow thy seed, and in the evening withhold not thine hand: for thou knowest not whether shall prosper, either this or that, or whether they both shall be alike good.

7. Truly the light is sweet, and a pleasant thing it is for the eyes to behold the sun: 8. But if a man live many years, and rejoice in them all; yet let him remember the days of darkness; for they shall be many. All that cometh is vanity.

9. Rejoice, O young man, in thy youth; and let thy heart cheer thee in the days of thy youth, and walk in the ways of thine heart, and in the sight of thine eyes: but know thou, that for all these things God will bring thee into judgment. 10. Therefore remove sorrow from thy heart, and put away evil from thy flesh: for childhood and youth are vanity.

12. 1. Remember now thy Creator in the days of thy youth, while the evil days come not, nor the years draw nigh, when thou shalt say, I have no pleasure in them; 2. While the sun, or the light, or the moon, or the stars, be not darkened, nor the clouds return after the rain: 3. In the day when the keepers of the house shall tremble, and the strong men shall bow themselves, and the grinders cease because they are few, and those that look out of the windows be darkened, 4. And the doors shall be shut in the streets, when the sound of the grinding is low, and he shall rise up at the voice of the bird, and all the daughters of musick shall be brought low; 5. Also when they shall be afraid of that which is high, and fears shall be in the way, and the almond tree shall flourish, and the grasshopper shall be a burden, and desire shall fail: because man goeth to his long home, and the mourners go about the streets: 6. Or ever the silver cord be loosed, or the golden bowl be broken, or the pitcher be broken at the fountain, or the wheel broken at the cistern. 7. Then shall the dust return to the earth as it was: and the spirit shall return unto God who gave it. 8. Vanity of vanities, saith the preacher; all is vanity.

The Fear of God is Utmost
9. And moreover, because the preacher was wise, he still taught the people knowledge; yea, he gave good heed, and sought out, and set in order many proverbs. 10. The preacher sought to find out acceptable words: and that which was written was upright, even words of truth.
11. The words of the wise are as goads, and as nails fastened by the masters of assemblies, which are given from one shepherd. 12. And further, by these, my son, be admonished: of making many books there is no end; and much study is a weariness of the flesh.
13. Let us hear the conclusion of the whole matter: Fear God, and keep his commandments: for this is the whole duty of man. 14. For God shall bring every work into judgment, with every secret thing, whether it be good, or whether it be evil.[54]

I am doing yoga, but it's still not good and I don't have a feeling that I want to do this regularly. This group, like others, has not decided yet whether to let me in.

Ronnie tells me to read John Bowlby because I find it difficult to part from people I spend time with.[55] When I was younger, I used to suffer from loneliness a lot. He says anxiety is a common reaction to being abandoned by someone we feel close to. Separation is a very different experience for the one who leaves than for the one who is left. This anxiety sometimes turns into anger, which starts with babies. All babies feel anger at being separated from their mother when they don't want to be separated. Anxiety may also come from the fear of blowing up with this anger, which is something that's not acceptable for adults. Masturbation may be the best way to relieve this anxiety. Ronnie believes men project the umbilical cord on our cock when we masturbate. When the boy child is playing with the umbilical cord in his mother's womb, it pulsates like an ejaculating cock in a man's hand. Surely, it also helps a woman to hold onto an ejaculating cock when she feels separation anxiety. Ronnie believes some people eat to relieve anxiety, others find a woman or man, anyone, just to have sex, others masturbate or drink. We have to do something that's pleasurable, and then we can turn anxiety into pleasure. He emphasises how crucial it is to allow ourselves to feel or think whatever we need to, and to be inquisitive. But we have to be careful with what feeling or thought we will transform into action. I always have the freedom to not eat when I want to eat, to not have sex when I want to have sex, or to not jerk off when I want to jerk off. I may have a feeling that I want to murder someone, but actually doing it is very different. Americans don't know this, Ronnie says. His idea is that by examining and getting to know the ways, desires, and emotions of our hearts, we can serve others with a similar heart. The more one allows one's emotions to flow freely, the more keenly and clearly one can feel these emotions in one's body. I tell him I had this impulse to squeeze my child's arm and to shake him. I noticed this impulse in my body, and I know that this is what my mother did to me. But I don't pass it on. Ronnie didn't have this experience. He wants to fight and thump people immediately. I tell him I saw Ballet Rambert, and I was so moved by their piece, "Tutti-frutti," that I almost started crying.[56] Your heart resonated with this music and dance, says Ronnie. When the heart resonates harmoniously, one starts crying.

I feel 17 or 18 years old with all my new books. One of Ronnie's tangles is that, if I don't know that I don't know, then I think I know. If I don't know that I know, then I think that I don't know. The earliest expression of this thought is in the Samaveda: if you think you know, then you don't know.[57] The other notion is that those who know, know that it is impossible to know. We talk about the tradition of Skeptics, about Husserl, the dialogues of Socrates, Montaigne, and an epigram of Chinese Taoist, Zhuang Zi.

Once, Zhuang Zhou dreamed he was a butterfly and fluttered about like a butterfly. He was contented and happy, not knowing he was Zhou! Suddenly, he woke up and found himself to be Zhou. It is not certain whether Zhou dreamed of changing into a butterfly or a butterfly dreamed of changing into Zhou. There must have been a demarcation between Zhou and a butterfly. This is called "transformation of things".[58]

We talk about Euripides[59]: how do I know that I am alive and not dead? Ronnie says the only thing stopping him from slitting his own neck is that no one is certain about anything. Pythia, the Oracle of Delphi, declared that Socrates was the wisest man, but Socrates himself evaluated this as follows:

but the truth is, O men of Athens, that God only is wise; and by his answer he intends to show that the wisdom of men is worth little or nothing; he is not speaking of Socrates, he is only using my name by way of illustration, as if he said, he, O men, is the wisest, who, like Socrates, knows that his wisdom is in truth worth nothing.[60]

The fruit of serious learning is wisdom, not knowledge. What is worth knowing? That we know very little and even that we don't know for certain. T.S. Eliot asks, "Where is the wisdom we have lost in knowledge? Where is the knowledge we have lost in information?"[61] We acquire knowledge from learning and education, while we gain wisdom from our daily experiences. Wisdom is a state of consciousness. Knowledge just sees facts and reality clearly, while wisdom is for making good decisions. But we have to be careful, says Ronnie, because undeserved skepticism is worse than pretending to know everything. In other words, if one constantly and almost automatically doubts everything, one will become boring and depressing. The heart cannot become skeptical, only the brain.

Francis asks, "Who isn't terrified of love?" We talk about Jonah, from the Bible, who receives the call, his calling, but he doesn't want to follow it. Francis believes that if one rejects one's calling it will poison one's heart.

Giorgio Agamben, whom I discovered years later, writes beautifully about our genius: "A Latin phrase perfectly expresses the secret relationship each person must maintain with his own Genius: indulgere genio. One must consent to Genius and abandon oneself to him; one must grant him everything he asks for, for his exigencies are our exigencies, his happiness our happiness. Even if his — our! — requirements seem unreasonable and capricious, it is best to accept them without argument. If in order to write you need — he needs! — a certain light-yellow paper, a certain special pen, a certain dim light shining from the left, it is useless to tell yourself that just any pen will do, that any paper and any light will suffice. If life is not worth living without that light blue linen shirt (for goodness' sake, not the white one with the collar of an office worker!), if without those long cigarettes with black paper you just don't see any reason to go on, then there's no point in repeating to yourself that these are no more than little manias, that now is the time to be over and done with them. In Latin, Genium suum defraudare, to defraud one's own genius, means to make one's life miserable, to cheat oneself, in Latin. But the life that turns away from death and responds without hesitation to the impetus of the genius that engendered it is called genialis, genial.[62]

I start reading one of the small books. It's tiny, and I bought it for only a pound. *Karma Yoga*, by Swami Vivekananda. According to him, we should work for the sake of working, not for the result. Work for working. Karma actually means work, and this is the yoga of work, not reincarnation or something like that. I like it! It is a weakness to think that anyone or anything depends on me, or that I could do good for anyone. This belief is the mother of all attachment. Attachment is the source of all pain. I like this idea, in the book, that we should inform our brain, our mind, that nobody in the universe depends on us. No beggar depends on your charity, no soul depends on your kindness, and no living entity needs your help. Nature doesn't stop for a moment because of you or without you. It carries on working even if a million of us disappear into the void. It's a privilege to be allowed to teach oneself through helping others. The great secrets are tiny things! All you need to do is practise it. Never say it is mine. I really like this book because by knowing that I am not needed, I can regain my freedom. From now on, I will never forget, not even for a moment, that I don't have to do anything. This is the most important book of my life!

Once, while driving home from the theatre with my wife, a truck almost crashed into us. It just missed, and we nearly died. The kids were at home with a babysitter. I pulled over to let my heartbeat settle down, and I had a momentary vision of us dying. I saw the children in a vacuum. But almost immediately, I sensed other people entering the vacuum and that the children didn't die of us not being there. They grow up differently but not necessarily worse. Suddenly, I felt incredibly free. I can never again say that I cannot do something because of my kids. It doesn't mean I can neglect them, but that I can't use them as an excuse when I don't want to do something. That's the truth.

Around New Year's Eve, I go visit Budapest and meet Gábor Karátson.[63] I buy corn on the cob for three forints, and it reminds me of my childhood. I read William Blake with Gábor. He reads Novalis for me. He is translating it from German into Hungarian as he reads it.

I am going back to London. I am leaving my beautiful motherland. The train is clickety clacking. It is cold, no light, no heating. It smells of sausages because I have a Yugoslavian family of five sleeping next to me. The man speaks a little Hungarian. He was looking for matches but he didn't have any forints. I gave him ten forints, but he couldn't find matches. The train window steamed

up from all the garlicky breaths. You can only see the scenery
from the corridor. Everything is bleak, grey and cold. It's getting

dark. The trees reach to the sky as if they were capillaries in the lungs of a huge animal. The earth breathes with them. Yugoslavian snoring. It was so good being home! It didn't take long. I've already forgotten the whole border-crossing chaos and aside from that, I had a wonderful time.

"No Smoking!" My seat is No. 62. The corridor is very busy. People are lugging bags around. Some stand outside having a smoke.

I spent a lot of time with Gábor, Szilvia, Dávid and János.[64] They are all special people. Why are our lives entwined together? Who are they to me? Who am I to them?

The train service is called Wiener Waltzer. It's late. I start meditating. I imagine or dream that I saw Szilvia's breast, but it went through a curious transformation and bits of turd came out of the nipple. An interesting confusion. It's too dark to write. I stop. I speak with Ronnie about this dream. I remember that in Hungarian you can say "to express" the breast. This reminds me of the word "expression". Words are coming, the mother's breast, mother's milk, mother tongue, vocabulary. I can see it bit by bit as it comes out of her breast.

Haya Oakley calls me to look after Collin in the shelter at 27 Shaftesbury Avenue. I only see Collin for a moment. His room is on the top of the stairs. All the windows are broken, there are bits of food and dirt on the floor, and old caked-on shit on the walls. The house is horrible. As I am walking around, everything smells of shit. Collin shits on the top landing, then kicks it down the stairs. He spends the whole night in his bed, wrapped in a blanket, and I am cleaning the place. He stays on his own upstairs; nobody goes there. I don't think Collin's environment even vaguely comes close to normalcy. This cannot be seen as resembling the womb. The whole house begs one to vandalise it, to become destructive, to not look after it, and it is so dirty and bad, you can only make it worse.

My relationship with the other is like a tightrope. I am dancing on this rope. I had the same feeling with my children. I can fall off the rope to the left or to the right; one side is neglect and the other is overbearing restriction and scrutiny, intrusiveness. One of the reasons Collin lost his mind was that he was controlled too much. He benefited from the neglect that surrounded him, and that his caretakers tolerated him. Other mad people need a different kind of environment. You can never know what kind of environment a living organism needs. If I want to love them, I really need to pay attention and try different things until I find the one that is best for them: more water, less water, more sunshine, less, lots of attention, company, or solitude and loneliness?

I am still vulnerable after my trip to Budapest. I have a sense that I am a link, that I need to connect things: Hungary with England, or my mother with my father. But I don't actually belong anywhere. It would be better to belong everywhere. Ronnie says I am looking better than ever and I start crying because I feel happy and sad at the same time. Ronnie says I am a lucky fellow: my desires are possible to fulfil within the framework of reality. Why could I not be the link who is appreciated by several cultures? Not letting go of my Hungarianness makes me a more interesting person. We talk about the origins of the word "nostalgia". It comes from the Greek word *nostos*, meaning return, homecoming, and *algeo*, which means feeling pain. This is the soft pain of longing for one's home. Until recently, it was called the Swiss disease because the soldiers of a Swiss army division died, while in Polish captivity, of desperately missing their mountains. It is an unusual kind of pain, very different from any other type of affliction caused by separation. The only thing one can do is to accept it, allow it and pay attention to it. One doesn't need to resist it. It takes a lot of energy to suppress something because the energy we expend to suppress it is compounded by the effort we make to ensure it doesn't crop up somehow. So, it takes double the energy. It is better to accept it.

I am talking with Jutta and she is irate because the cleaner didn't come on time. I ask her whether Ronnie helps with the chores. Jutta says she doesn't expect him to. It wouldn't be possible anyway. He does his job so well; it is better he just does that. Jutta likes it when everything is tidy. Ronnie did the dishes once or twice, but it wasn't much good. He couldn't do it to satisfy Jutta's standards. When they visited Sri Lanka, he left Jutta on her own for weeks because it was his trip, not their trip. It's not easy living with a dominant character. She says she would constantly feel angry and poisoned if she resented Ronnie or those who visit him. She accepts Ronnie as the better person.

I am at Haya's seminar. I tell her that, two weeks ago, I had a dream about Collin's shit, and that I have read Wolf Wolfensberger, who writes about normalising environments.[65] He says that the environment shapes one's actions. We should be careful with the kind of environment we leave Collin in. Haya says Collin is frightened by warmth, he wants cold, and he wants a cold draft whistling through his room. If this is what he wants, we let him have it. He doesn't just break the window again and again when we repair it, he rips out the shutters as well. Haya thinks it is important that he is allowed to do this. Collin keeps doing this as if he wanted to break out of his foetal caul. Only Collin lives in this house now. Everyone else is angry with him because he is very inconsiderate, but he didn't get kicked out. Everyone went somewhere else, temporarily. Haya feels responsible because she took him there. I think it is much harder to form a community around Collin than to integrate him into an already-working community. As far as I can see, there is no working, mature community here. Haya says that Collin always eats from the same place on the floor, and whatever he puts into his mouth, it has to touch the ground first. He doesn't just pee and poo on the floor, he spills or splatters anything that can be spilled, including two-thirds of all the food and drink he has. Haya thinks we should play with this. If Collin thinks the floor is the placenta, let's give him three things to eat but take two back immediately. She thinks Collin might eat all of the one thing left, instead of throwing away two-thirds of it.

What a miracle! She tried it and it worked. Collin later came to his senses. He was cured and left the shelter, but it took another year.

Hugh Crawford is reading Ivan Illich's new book, *Medical Nemesis*, and he feels the situation is hopeless.[66] It will have to be started all over again: the shelter, the world, and everything. He started doing yoga when he felt his organs and body begin to decline, as he just sat in his office all day. Ronnie also talks about Illich. He really respects and enjoys the new book.

Seven of us meet at Ronnie's in the evening for a seminar. The topic is preparations for a new group that Ronnie wants to start. It's a practical therapy workshop. He only wants to direct it and the seven of us, his team, will do everything. He envisions four circles. The first, or inner circle, would be the eight of us. In the second circle are those who are ready to do something. In the third circle are those who are not ready yet but want to do something. And in the fourth circle are those who don't want to do anything; they just want to be onlookers. Ronnie thinks we need an audience to make the whole thing more dramatic. Having an audience, having outside attention, will make what's happening inside the circle hotter. Attention boils things. He thinks we need drama. He is more interested in exercises that don't need words than those that require speaking. So there is no discussion, no theory, no sharing circle or such formalised bullshit, only the exercises. Everyone can take their experiences home and do what they want with them. Ronnie is exemplary in looking after himself. In the group, he fights for what he wants and runs away from what he doesn't want. He even fell asleep once, after whispering in my ear and asking me, as his co-leader, whether it would bother me. He expects the same from everyone in the group. If one doesn't want to take part in a particular thing, one can leave and re-enter as one wants. There is no talking people into things and no force. Zero coercion, zero persuasion

– invitation only. The members of the group all study in the Philadelphia Association and everyone has their own therapist. If the workshop starts a process in somebody, they can discuss it with their own therapist.

I sit in for a therapy session and Ronnie's patient doesn't mind. He is a 35-year-old Swiss photographer and businessman named Christian. He wants to get into one of the shelters, and Ronnie just gives him directions: Christian can see him, or if he wants, he can go to the shelter without therapy. Christian seems nervous and hyperactive. He pulls out various things from his briefcase and is showing Ronnie letters, poems, books and discharge reports. A while back, he was diagnosed with manic depression. He used to take lithium, but one day he flushed all the medication down the toilet. This was a good few months ago and now he is trying to live without medication.

It's the weekend, so there is no one in London except me. Christian loses his mind and freaks out. None of the shelters accepts him, no one can look after him, so I have to get a taxi and take him to the hospital. I feel really guilty. I think our job is to prevent people from ending up in hospital but there is nothing I can do for him. Later, I call the psychiatrist to find out what's happening. He says Christian is under observation, but they are not sure whether he is psychotic or manic.

Christian got a bed in a room with a big black guy who instantly fell in love with him. He approached him eagerly, which terrified Christian, and he hid under the duvet. But the big black man lifted up the bed and tipped him out. Within a few hours, Christian manages to convince the psychiatrist that he is well and wants to go home to Switzerland. They let him go. Well, this is great.

I tell Ronnie what happened and how I don't understand myself. I can be gentle with some people but Christian just made me want to kick him in the arse and shake him. I had no empathy for him. Ronnie is smiling. One's own experiences are reliable instruments to figure out the other person. If I experience tenderness, that probably means the other person is regressing, they are actually becoming little and I empathise with that. On the other hand, if someone just pretends to be little but they are being wilful, which is a synonym for madness, then one has to snap at them and tell them to come off it. I should just trust my experiences and not criticise myself.

Silent Evening Psalm, by Attila József

Oh, Lord, I can't hammer your glory into rhymes.
I recite my psalm with humble lips.
But if You'd rather not, don't listen to my words.

I know grass turns green, but I don't understand why and for whom.
I feel I love, but I don't yet know whose mouth my lips will burn.
I hear the wind blowing, but I don't know why it blows, when I feel gloomy.
But don't mind my words if You don't like them.

Just simply, primitively I'd like to tell You now that I am,
and I'm here and admire you, but I don't understand You.

For You don't need our admiration and psalming about.
For the loud and unending appeals may hurt Your ears.
For we can do nothing but pray, abase ourselves and beg.

I'm your humble slave, who You can give away even to Hell.
Your realm is infinite and You are mighty, strong and eternal.
Oh, Lord, give my tiny little humble self to me.

But if you'd rather not, don't listen to my words.[67]

I say this to myself often…

Ronnie tells me about his morning patient, a 60-year-old Pakistani man, a former ambassador, who has been looking for the
truth for 50 years. He meditates regularly and now he has some
buzzing sound, some vibration in his head, like a small whirlpool
of sound. It disturbs him and he is unable to control it. Ronnie
asks me if I think it could be treated with hypnosis. The man is
accepting, open to influences, and as Ronnie puts his hand on
his head, he says that he can feel the energy emanating from
Ronnie's hand. He is a dream acupuncture patient. Ronnie gives
him tuning forks to vibrate on his head. Ronnie and I talk about
how the man is actually having an erection in his head; the blood
is rushing there instead of his genitals.

Observation: Ronnie gives himself to every one of his patients.
He thinks about them like he thinks about himself and tries everything that could work. Ronnie has sent another patient to
Francis. The man experiences himself as if he had been twisted
180 degrees. He didn't say he could see what was behind him

but he has this constant sense of being twisted, of being turned around. Francis has tried all sorts of things, like hypnosis and massage, but nothing has helped. Ronnie thought maybe he could try LSD but he is worried that the man might not be strong and healthy enough. After the LSD he might become even more twisted and that would be dangerous. Francis tells us a story about a Zen master who took LSD in the company of his high-class Western disciples. He ended up having a huge erection, jerked off two or three times, and was moaning that he needed his wife and one of his good friends. Francis thinks the strict and hard spiritual practice pushed sexuality aside but LSD brought everything back to the centre. It is always dangerous to disturb the balance. The master said he would have to start everything all over again.

I have an opportunity now to stay in London for good. My practice is becoming more popular and lucrative and we have enough money to live here. Still, we decide to go home. I talk with Ronnie about my fear. I am not sure whether my decision to move back to Vancouver in June is a real decision that will benefit me, or if it is a defence mechanism to save me from having to go deeper, having to learn more. As I am talking, I make a slip. I want to say "when my money runs out", but I say "when my Ronnie muns out", instead. "Ronnie" instead of "money". Well, brilliant. Ronnie is silent and doesn't say a word. Then he says that this is my decision. He can see the advantages of both leaving and staying.

I still think it was a good decision because I had grown up by then and needed to try my own wings.

I tell him about the friction with my wife. It's about housework. Meredith doesn't make any money and I don't do any housework, but we constantly argue about it. Ronnie says his way of solving this problem with Jutta is by trying to make enough money so Jutta doesn't have to do everything herself. She can have a cleaning lady, and they can go out for meals. Ronnie won't do the dishes or clean the house, that's for sure.

Kevin, a 28-year-old, comes to see Ronnie for his first session. He has been going through therapists since he was 16. He's had nineteen of them so far, and he has taken tons of medications and even had electroshocks. He starts off by saying that coming here is like going to see the Pope. He talks very loudly. He has a terrible stutter, and vowels catch his tongue. He is frustrated, and he frustrates us. Ronnie is very patient. He listens very attentively and, at the end, he talks about how therapy can bring light to darkness. Ronnie tells a Sufi tale about Nasreddin Hodja:

Hodja lost a ring somewhere in his house. He looked for it but didn't find it anywhere, so he went outside and continued looking in front of the door. His neighbour asked him what he was looking for. When he understood that Hodja was looking for a ring he had lost in the house, he asked, "Why are you looking outdoors then?" "Well, it's too dark indoors. I can see better in this light."[68]

When Kevin leaves, Ronnie says the boy is not ready for therapy yet. He still wants someone to do something to him, to cure him. He is not present yet and he doesn't understand that he has to find his own path because nobody can solve his existential situation. Ronnie wouldn't mind if Kevin sees me for sessions because I still have the energy to accompany him until he becomes mature enough to start therapy. Of course, what happens before is also therapy but, long term, Ronnie doesn't have the patience for this anymore. First, Kevin would need to have experiences and see connections that he has avoided so far. He doesn't link things together at all. He is like a virgin with no knowledge of sex. He talks about himself in an impersonal theoretical way and he has no insights. We agree that Kevin will see me.

I am reading Freud about melancholy and narcissism.[69] I ponder whether this is what I am suffering from, whether my neurosis is narcissistic. According to Freud, those in this category don't fall into transference, and well, that's true. I respect Ronnie but there is not much transference in that. Of course, I question that as well. Maybe there is a lot of transference, but I can't see it? I always get really confused when I read Freud. What would he have said about me? He says narcissism is incurable. Fuck off, then. I had a supervisor at Simon Fraser University. He was the supervisor of my PhD thesis and when I went to see him in his office to discuss something, he leaned back in his chair, folded his hands behind his head, and looked in my direction but somehow not at me. It was an odd feeling. When I stood up, I saw that there was a mirror behind me, and he was looking at himself the whole time. Well, that is narcissism.

It seems to me that Ronnie is not so much interested in me, but in his own experiences while being with me. This may be narcissism, too, but I don't know whether it is possible to enjoy someone in any other way than enjoying one's own experiences in that person's company. But how do I know what is happening with the other person? If a man is terrified of not having an erection when he has sex with a woman, if he starts being fearful when he is with a woman, then he watches himself and pays attention to whether his cock is getting hard instead of smelling, tasting, touching, admiring, embracing, enjoying and worshipping the woman. He is not lost in the woman but is taken with whether his cock is getting hard. He is absorbed in himself. He is paying attention to his own cock. But if God wanted us to be in control, he would have made the penis out of muscle. It is not made of muscle for a reason. He has to pay attention to the other person, not himself. That will lift him out of his narcissism.

Ronnie included some of the dreams I told him in his book. I am of two minds about this. On one hand, it's great that he paid attention and found what I said so interesting; on the other hand, what if he just fucking used me and only cares about the dreams, not me?

The Epilogue of the Lyric Poet, by Mihály Babits

Compelled to be the hero of my verse,
the first and last in every song I write,
I long to shape in them the universe,
but naught beyond myself comes into my sight.

There's naught but me: such thoughts I start to nurse;
if there is, God alone can get it right.
A blind nut shut in shell: this is my curse –
To await being cracked in hateful night.

To break my magic ring I try in vain.
Only my arrow pierces it: desire —
though I know well my hopes will shrink by half.

Prison for my own self I must remain,
being subject and object, son and sire,
being, alas, both omega and alpha.[70]

I am at Heaton's seminar. The topic is whether it is possible to speak about transcendental experiences like God. What does it mean to experience God? What kind of experience is it to be with God or to be God? Tibetan monks and lamas study logic for years before they start meditating. Heaton thinks that first one has to study language. Logic is to make sure language can't pull the wool over our eyes. It is easy to say things and easy to create nonsense. There are many words, like "God", "goodness", "justice", and it is possible that they are all one and the same. According to Wittgenstein, we need nonsense because there is no sense. You can say "go and find the book" or "go and find God". They sound the same. Grammatically, it is the same thing, and language suggests that, if you can manage the first one, you can also accomplish the second. But there is a huge difference, says Wittgenstein. The first instruction is finished when you have the book in your hand but the second one never ends. "I want to be good-looking" or "I want to be good". The grammar and structure are the same but the experience is very different. So-called humanistic psychologists don't seem to be aware of this linguistic problem and they say a lot of crazy things. "Know your times tables!" "Know thyself!" "Develop your knowledge!" "Develop your personality!" A load of nonsense! Heaton thinks transcendence is beyond psychology and logic is useful to help us avoid and steer clear of non sequiturs or wrong conclusions. Husserl and Wittgenstein are both deeply interested in logic: how does one express reality? How does one say what is true, and say as much as needed, without saying too much or too little? In this way, what we say and what exists in the world will concur and we can map the world accurately. Heaton gives these examples:

Mary is pretty.
You're going to marry Mary.
You're going to marry someone pretty. – True.

Someone is pretty.
You're going to marry someone.
You're going to marry a pretty woman. – False.

It's wonderful that we have logic and mathematics. Albert Einstein writes an equation and suddenly the world reflects the equation and the equation reflects the world. How is it possible that we live in such a logical, mathematical world? Heaton says it is only possible because the human mind from which, and with which, we express ourselves, and which came up with mathematics and logic is actually one with the universe. Being surprised by this is due to the misconception that the mind is not the world. Well, this is the Cartesian error that separates the mind from everything else. But if we accept the mind as the mapping of the universe, it doesn't sound as outlandish any more. Why could it not be like that, Heaton asks? An ocean in a drop. The universe in the mind. If I am the universe, then everything I dream up is dreamed up by the universe. What can we find, and what can we not find? What can we help with, and what can we not help with? What can we demonstrate or teach, and what can we not? And what is the logic behind it all? Heaton explains that you can't give metaphysical directions to enlightenment because it is very different from showing the way to a cathedral. If we don't think this through, we get confused and start talking bullshit. "Follow me, I'll take you to the cathedral." That's fine. But "follow me, I'll take you to enlightenment"? That's bullshit. Looking for a colour is different than looking for a smell and different than looking for the centre of physical pain.

I talk with Francis a lot about shamans, their habits, characteristics, and about what shamanic illness is. He gives me a task: I have to carefully think about what is common in these five people: Huxley, Laing, Redler, Crawford and Heaton. Francis toys with the idea that all five men are shamans.

Huxley later wrote a major article about shamanism and Laing, which I have included in this book. He makes it clear that Laing wasn't a shaman, in the strict sense of the term, because he was doing something very different. He functioned differently from shamans. In his discussion with me, Francis was more playing with the word. He used it as a metaphor and he had me play with it, too. Around this time, I was studying anthropology and shamanism quite deeply. I had just read Francis's book, *The Way of the Sacred*. Olga Nagy's book, *Heroes, Cheaters, Devils*, is a brilliant book about the shaman, as is Kilton Stewart's book,

Pygmies and Dream Giants.[71] If one is interested in the subject, these books are a great start. I came across Sámuel Diószegi's books about Siberian shamans later on, when I was writing *Son of the Brown Cow* with Dorottya Büky.[72] Siberian shamans leave their body, ascend the world tree and attempt to retrieve, fight for, the lost soul of their patient. Voodoo priests vacate themselves and allow various spirits to take possession of them, speaking and acting through them for the benefit of the afflicted. What is certain is that shamans give themselves up to the spirit of the situation. That is true about Laing. And the rest, who knows?

I am reading Mircea Eliade's book about shamanism.[73]

Crawford's shelter is a shaman's theatre. Every shaman likes the theatre. Ronnie is not interested in the work of other shamans and that's also typical of shamans. Brazilian shamans are totally disinterested in each other. They couldn't care less. According to Carlos Castaneda, wizards and shamans only have one working eye. Francis and I can both only really see with one eye. This would indicate that I am a shaman, too. Ronnie is simultaneously a rogue and a very kind-hearted person. This places everyone in a double bind. Shamans often put people in a double bind, just like Zen masters with the koan because they attract and repel at the same time. Shamans hold their heads high, even physically. By lifting your nose, you can balance your head on your neck without having to use the shoulder muscles. Francis thinks my head hanging down reflects servility. I should hold my head higher. And Francis thinks Ronnie expects others to join his

215

fun, his enjoyment, but he never joins theirs. When he plays the piano, he expects others to listen enthusiastically but he won't listen to anyone else. And Ronnie is an expert at being silent. When he is silent, everyone becomes anxious. Francis has not yet asked Ronnie about what he does when he is silent. When Ronnie opens the door to let someone in, it's a curious mixture of a kind-hearted warm welcome and a suspicious, wary reticence. Francis gave Ronnie a gift of a beautiful Buddha hand and shows me what he got from Ronnie: a shitty walking stick. The wood has rotted away and it's a useless, worthless piece of scrap, you can't even burn it. He wouldn't want to be seen with it, that's for sure. He is laughing it off but it is a fact that Ronnie looks down on everyone. He only has respect for one or two people, here and there. He likes to duel and if you can stand your ground, he'll respect you; otherwise, he doesn't give a shit. The double bind spins you around – yes, no, yes, no, yes, no. The spin will sometimes provide enough force to launch you into space like a rocket.

After this, I spin over to Ronnie. I tell him, because I am still living in Freudian terminology, how much transference I am capable of because I may be too narcissistic. He says when he used to read Freud, he didn't accept the Freudian categories but created his own. Whatever wasn't corroborated by his own experiences, he changed.

I tell him how it is difficult to decide when to move back to Vancouver. It hurts to think about it. He says there is no need to do it that way. The treatment is to be one hundred percent present in every moment and then you don't have time to suffer.

He finds a poem by Kathleen Raine and reads it out to me.[74] You can love without being attached. Departure is painful if you are attached, because then the glue of attachment has to break, but if there is no attachment, you can make a break without suffering. He met a 100-year-old saint in India and could ask him only one question: "How to live truly?" "Transform your heart into the sun and shine on everyone equally." To the sun, it doesn't matter if there are some idiots who hide from its heat and light.

I feel stronger than ever before. I think I am not even neurotic, any longer. Sometimes it still seems I can't connect to things or people and I don't know where I could fit myself in to have self-confidence and energy. I am still afraid to say everything that's on my mind. If I stood before a firing squad, I think I would collapse before they fired. Ronnie just says that our whole environment, our entire society, is estranged and switched off. He normalises my crap.

I haven't got a secret chart
to get me to the heart of this
or any other matter.[75]

Before leaving, I somehow feel the need to ask Ronnie to bless me. He puts his hand on my head and strokes my hair gently. There is a party at Mina's. Ronnie is there and plays the piano from 11 till half-past 12, one song after the other, and each one is supposed to be the last one. The taxi has to wait for him until he finishes. He plays "My Melancholy Baby" and "Bye Bye Blackbird" several times because he knows I'll leave soon. He plays songs from *Black Orpheus* and then plays Bach with Leon.

Francis hugs and kisses me. Ronnie too. We say our goodbyes.
Then Mina, Arthur, Mel, Michael, Peter, Leon, David, Haya,
Dodo, Stef, Margo, Ron, Paul…

After spending a year together, I got these two letters from R.D.
Laing and Francis Huxley as a certificate of achievement or diploma.

For me, this was my initiation: The boy turned into a man.

R.D. Laing   65a Belsize Park Gardens London N.W.3 01-586-164(

June 20, 1975

To whom it may concern:

During 1974/75, Andrew Feldmar spent ten months
in analysis with me, and I supervised his clinical
practice.

He has completed his apprenticeship to my
satisfaction, and I consider him my associate.

He is a psychotherapist whose skill, judgement
and understanding I trust.

R. D. Laing, M.B., Ch.B., D.P.M.
Chairman - Philadelphia Association
Fellow - Royal Society of Medicine

                                                    sise Park Gardens
                                                    a N.W.3.

                                                    6.75

To whom it may concern:

   During 1974/75, Andrew Feldmar attended my seminars given within
the Study Programme of the Philadelphia Association, and for six
months we have met weekly to discuss readings, ideas and experiences
from the general areas of Anthropology, Psychoanalysis, Religion,
Myth and Literature, with special emphasis on shamanism, dreams,
symbolism and healing.

   I judge him capable of organising and carrying out research in
a scholarly and creative manner. I also recommend him as a sensitive
and insightful teacher; and, in short, consider him my friend, and
associate.

                                    Francis Huxley

                                    Francis Huxley

A CONVERSATION
WITH R.D. LAING

During 1974–75, when I spent a year in London, England, working with R.D. Laing, in addition to being in analysis with him, he also supervised my practice. I thoroughly immersed myself in the life of the Philadelphia Association, a network of households that provided asylum for profoundly disturbed people.

In May of 1979, I visited Ronnie Laing again, and after several discussions, he agreed to a taped interview. At the last minute, Dr Leon Redler joined us in Ronnie's spacious consulting room. Leon had been Ronnie's associate since the days of Kingsley Hall (1965). The three of us spent two and a half hours talking, drinking and occasionally listening to Adam, Ronnie's 12-year-old son, practising Bach on the piano upstairs, where the Laings lived.

The following is a transcription of our talk. Every time I read it, I recollect the warmth, hospitality and friendship that filled the room.

LOVE

Andrew Feldmár: To begin with, I'd like to focus on your use of the concept of love or loving.

You use it often. On the dust jacket of *The Facts of Life*, for instance, you say, "Without the experience of love, or at least a memory of it, or a memory of a hallucination of it, life is not worth living."[1] Recently, I read a definition of love by Ashley Montagu which is quite specific.[2] He figures that it has real survival value and that it has a real genetic basis. I have never heard you talk about what you mean by love when you talk about it.

R.D. Laing: It would be fitting to consider a number of the different sorts of things that are often covered by the same word, and the initial semantic problem that the same word can mean different things and different words might mean the same thing. I'm *not* talking about desire. That's the most important distinction. I'm *not* talking about any form of desire, from the Buddhist sense to the Sanskrit sense, or as it is used in other places, as, for example, it crops up in psychoanalytic theory as libido. It becomes difficult, of course, with Freud, where he, in a later paper, sees a very close affinity, if not an identity, between his notion of libido and what he calls "Platonic love". The love that I'm referring to is the same as the love referred to by St Paul in Corinthians as *charity*. There have been a number of attempts to define love in that sense. It finds a classical expression in St Thomas Aquinas, for whom love consisted in the knowing of that which is, in its isness.[3]

This obviously entails letting be, entails seeing and wanting it to be and cherishing it for itself as it is. Any amplification alluding to love by a formula like that becomes extremely subtle, if not confused, because if love has something to do with a compassionate letting be, without attachment, without desire, without any self-serving in it, there is a problem with the confrontation of love and evil. To indicate that I'm not talking about the term as usually applied in terms of desire or in terms of affect (i.e., like or dislike), I could imagine the emotion of hatred being an expression of love.

AF: Knowing, then, is very intimately connected to loving.

RDL: Aquinas, summarising a whole tradition, said that there is no knowledge without love.[4] You can't know except through the medium of love. Love is the only way through which knowledge can become apparent or manifest. All knowledge is predicated upon love, so if there is knowledge, there must be love, and without love, there is no knowledge. This basic epistemology seems to be what's been cut across by the project of natural science that proposes we can know *all* we are, in fact we are going to know, by eliminating love from the negotiation. No love enters into the relationship between the investigating scientist and their object of inquiry. They think they can maximise their scientific knowledge, their tautology, the more they eliminate any consideration for what they are looking at. They can do anything they like to it, mess around with it as much as they like, destroy it, create it even, totally lovelessly, maybe with a certain amount of desire but without any concern or consideration or regard for the thing in itself.

AF: In an old play by George Chapman, called *All Fools*, the character Valerio says this about love:

I tell thee, Love is Nature's second Sun,
Causing a spring of virtues where he shines;
And as without the Sun, the World's great eye,

All colours, beauties, both of Art and Nature,
Are given in vain to men; so without Love
All beauties bred in women are in vain,
All virtues born in men lie buried;
For Love informs them as the Sun doth colours;
And as the Sun, reflecting his warm beams,
Against the earth, begets all fruits and flowers,
So Love, fair shining in the inward man,
Brings forth in him the honourable fruits
Of Valour, wit, virtue and haughty thoughts,
Brave resolution: and divine discourse:
Oh, 'tis the Paradise, the heaven of earth.[5]

RDL: Nice.

THERAPY

AF: Gurdjieff was described to have brutal relationships with his disciples. Could that still be an expression of love?

RDL: Ah, well, the word "brutal" is rather *extreme*. One wonders whether anything that we would like to reserve for the term "brutal" could be an expression of love. However, it's certainly obvious that love can take many forms of expression that might *look* brutal or be physically quite harsh. I mean, the Japanese system of hitting a pupil with a stick under certain circumstances doesn't seem to me to preclude, in any way, love. It depends how it is done. If there is a bit of spite behind it, and the person's getting off on it, but of course. I think that

226

all the numerous disciplines that people observe in different parts of the world, in different traditions, under different, very often individual, gurus or teachers are all subsumed into the overall context of ultimate love, peace and harmonisation. These practices occur within a context of acceptance. So, I think that's where the reconciliation between the terms of this contradiction lies. I don't think it's necessarily the most loving thing to never lose one's temper, never get angry, never tell someone, even quite viciously, some hard truths they could do with hearing for their own self-protection.

AF: Do you think that is what Winnicott meant in his article on the necessity of the expression of hatred?

RDL: "Hate in The Counter-Transference"?

AF: Yes.

RDL: He certainly referred to that paper when I was in supervision with him. He regarded the emotions that occur to one as *not* within one's control. He didn't believe that there was an ideal state of one's feelings being perfectly analysed out of one. He didn't equate feelings with neurotic symptoms. It is no credit, in my book, to an enlightened analyst that he impassively hears all the stuff that is put to him, sometimes quite personally challenging, and never feels anything. All feelings bifurcate, really, into love or hatred. We may want more or less of a feeling; we may want to stop it or let it continue; we may want to annul it, erase it or destroy it. One of the ways we have, which may be completely primitive, in our basic programme of dealing with a situation that we don't like is that we either remove ourselves from it or we can attempt to change the situation. One way we can change the situation, if we can't rearrange it, is to erase one element or some elements of it. It's killing, it's murdering, it's rubbing out. You can rub a person out, you can rub a thought out, you can rub a memory out, and if you can't rub the perceptions out, you might have to rub the stimulus out that is causing the unwanted input. Destroy the source of input if you can't deny or repress it. "Kill it!" It seems a very logical thing to do. Some people seem, however, to derive an unfortunate degree of erotic satisfaction out of doing that. There has been a merging, as Freud describes, with Eros in the service of Thanatos. Such people even seek out opportunities in order to employ that manoeuvre and act with glee at the chance of it coming their way. It is the opposite of general benevolence.

AF: Paul Goodman once wrote that he used to get erections when reading Freud.[6] Some of the ideas excited him so much, he got erotic pleasure out of them. There seems, then, to exist the opposite kind of erotic pleasure that derives from suppressing thoughts like that. One can get very excited by wiping out insights and people.

You have also worked with W.R. Bion. He recommends that a therapist should be in a "zero state" when working. Do you think that Bion is referring to an emotionless, memoryless state?

RDL: It's a state in which zero is being recorded. There are no presentations to the mind. There are no *darstellen*.[7] There are no, as Freud called them, "representations", although the mind is, of course, receiving. Strictly speaking, I would think, if you were in Bion's zero state and someone came through the door, someone you have been seeing five times a week for five years, you wouldn't recognise them. You would have to look at everything very carefully and think very hard, starting from scratch, before you knew what anything was. You can get into states like that in meditation.

AF: In zazen, for instance.

RDL: Yes, quite. Waking up from sleep, sometimes there might be a lapse of some time before one's reality orientation comes back. I don't think that Bion has quite managed to express what I imagine he is trying to say. He is a man of extremes. He was one of my instructors at the Psychoanalytic Society when I was in training. I didn't have any personal one-to-one supervision with him but I was in a number of his theoretical/clinical seminars. I had already published a paper using Bion-esque methods of pairing in psychoanalytic groups. I also met him socially. He told me at that time, that when he was working with his grid, he never made an interpretation intuitively, right off.[8] He never said anything for the first 40 minutes and then he summarised it all in his mind. He found a common group theme. He saw the different mechanisms of defence and what the basic catastrophe was that was being avoided by this rather than that. Then he made a completely formed interpretation. When he was doing it in a group, he made a group interpretation, then he addressed himself to individuals. He couched his words in rich body language, so you know just exactly who was putting whose penis up whose anus, you see. So, at that time, he was very far from any zero state. I imagine that he nearly drove himself out of his mind, formulating such exacting interpretations a number of hours every day, so after a while, he probably cultivated a sort of opposite procedure of presuppositionless coasting along, just letting anything appear

to him without naming it, labelling it, or without any conscious effort to connect it or anything. Taken to an extreme,
I don't see how you can understand even a sentence, because
you have to remember at least about a minute in order to put
any coherent unit of meaning together. I imagine the only way
one could understand what he is really after would be to have
a conversation with him.

AF: I have compared Gurdjieff's "way of blame", a harsher way
of being with people, to the Palo Alto School of Brief Therapy. Fisch, Weakland and Watzlawick feel that what they are
doing is very much like the clever stratagems of a Zen teacher.
When I worked with them, however, it didn't seem to me to
be a very loving way of being with people.[9]

RDL: I touched into all that maybe about 15 or 16 years ago.
You've really got to be in the mood for it. You've got to be
right in there. I think it would be a bit of an impertinence to
pronounce that one can't do that sort of short therapy lovingly.
It obviously lends itself to the worst sort of manipulative people. But I don't know whether one require that all therapists
should be saints or near-saints. If they are not, they must be
putting their numbers on people to a greater or lesser extent.
Is brief therapy a way that inevitably entails putting one's
own numbers on people, and is it essentially a transgression
on other people's lives so that it's perverted in its roots and
couldn't possibly yield very much but more confusion? Or is
it, as they say, a skilful means to jolt people out of their action
routines with each other, and awaken them to what they are
doing? By seeing, for instance, someone else behaving as they
have behaved, on the basis of a behavioural prescription that

someone has concocted: "The next time he comes on this way, instead of behaving complementary to him, behave symmetrically!" Well, I really don't know. I would hate to see it taken up institutionally by the social workers. It seems to me unteachable. It's like the subtle levels of a Zen master. Their reaction to their disciples is conditioned entirely by where they are at, by who they essentially are. To proliferate these techniques indiscriminately does make one feel that it's a giving of very dangerous toys to people, some of whom must be children, whatever their professional status is. Now, that's a bit alarming! To think of letting them loose on the population at large!

FORMS

AF: Reading your sonnets, I was thinking that you picked a very exacting form.[10] Your description of the basic essentials of therapy (a reliable time and place and two people coming together) seems to be a description of *form*. Do you find certain forms more conducive to bringing about what's desirable than other forms? You could decide the form, both in psychotherapy and in writing, before the content comes, couldn't you?

RDL: No, certainly I can only say it isn't like that. Suppose we were to try to make that distinction between morphology and content in biology, say, in terms of our own bodies. How can you describe what you would call content without implying the context all the time in the bare description of the content? Is the hand the content of the form of a limb? My left upper limb is made up of these: hand, lower arm and upper arm. You can break down what the hand is made up of, down to its most ultimately describable units, each of which has got no meaning without the arm context, which in a sense defines them.

The property of an element of any artistic unity is surely a function of the context, which I can't distinguish from form. Take the old basic definition of quality and quantity in music. The pitch of a note, say, is given the name of gamma, or call it G. Well, the quantity which is its abstract pitch has got absolutely no meaning of any kind whatever, without finding its context within a tune or composition, a musical context which immediately defines its qualitative relationship to the tonal region in which it is located. So, you can't take a phrase or line out of a sonnet and put it into a limerick, or take the abstract cask of a sonnet form and then fill it up. It's *not* that of a pint of wine to a bottle.

The original sense of sonnets was that a sonnet is a sigh. I think it's related to a breath. Most sonnets have the form of a breath of thought that goes out, goes in, and then turns around in the middle and reverses its movement, sometimes coming back in a sort of circular or spiral form, but it is always an out-and-in or an in-and-out breath.

AF: I find you are, specifically, very clear about forms. If you and I agree on some kind of a form and then one of us transgresses it, that transgression is likely to generate shame. I think you're very good at defining the boundaries of a situation, and that gives one the freedom to operate within it.

RDL: If you're dancing a tango, you can't suddenly dance a quickstep, or a waltz, so?

AF: Well, I guess what I'm asking you is: are you drawn to certain forms because they are more productive or better than others?

RDL: Oh, definitely, as I'm sure you are too. One doesn't want to be misunderstood in talking about form, forms that suit oneself, to suddenly be prescribing forms for everyone else. Because I happen to write sonnets, I'm not saying that everyone should start writing sonnets…

And that's what I'm accused of! I've been accused of that all my life by people who say I set a bad example. I've always, I think, avoided without difficulty prescribing what I find good for me at one time; it may not even be good for *me* at another time.

AF: Would you say that you *do* set an example, but on a higher logical level, i.e., it's a good idea for people to find their *own* form?

RDL: Of course! It's quite useful for Andrew to remind us of these elementary propositions which one is inclined to take for granted. It never, ever would have occurred to me that there is any way of arriving at form that wasn't one's own form. I mean, how can I impose my form on anyone else?! You would never dream of that, would you?

AF: Well, it happens often enough!

RDL: What state of mind must one be in to think one can take over someone else's form because they're grooving in that form! It's like watching a flower unfolding from itself into a form and to think you can suddenly take that form and wear it like clothes.

AF: Yes, but it happens: in psychoanalytic training, the form of the couch seems mandatory.

RDL: When I, as a child, was learning music, I wasn't going to argue with Mozart and Schubert about the form of a sonata.

I'll learn the sonata form gladly, and learn to write in sonata form to exercise myself. I won't say that that form of education is everyone's way or form of being musically educated, but I've no objection to that for myself. Most people who write in their own form have apprenticed themselves by their own choice to expend a lot of practice, practising this and that sort of thing, this and that sort of form. It's a great advantage that people have discovered pitches and *do, re, mi, fa, so, la, ti, do*'s and major and minor scales, and God knows how many modes and combinations of tones and quarter-tones. I am very glad to be alive within a ripe cultural tradition where many forms of expression have been explored deeply and even mathematically.

The people who think they're going to say anything to anyone by being "free spirits", in the sense that they're not going to assimilate these forms, will be disappointed. You take your chances that you're not going to be assimilated by tradition. If you haven't got the internal creative resilience to go through all these forms and master them, before going beyond them, then you just get silted down among them, and you go down under.

I can think of a number of different forms in which children can be brought up, but the family, as a social form, which is happy, is still a very nice form of life…

AF: What about open marriages, group marriages and other different kinds of living arrangements?

RDL: I don't see, I don't feel any internal necessity to say that, just because one form has been tried and proved to be a good form for some and for oneself during a certain stage of one's life, that other forms aren't feasible for oneself and for other people by their own witness. I'm not going to say someone is a liar if they live in a communal, sexual adult-and-child situation and find it delightful and happy and fine. Absolutely fine with me. I don't know of any spiritual tradition that, in its most fundamental statements, condemns any such forms out of hand.

TRANSFORMATIONS

AF: Once, you and I talked about transformations of experience. I often wonder when you or I analyse somebody's stated experience, in terms of whether it's a true, primary experience or a transformation of a primary experience, I wonder what guidelines you have for rolling back a series of transformations. It seems to be a very tenuous, very difficult process. I talked to you once about one of my patients who seemed to be turned on by his wife coming home telling him that she had just slept with another man. He felt delighted to think that there were still traces of another man inside his wife. I think you mentioned that that could be a transformation of a basic jealous experience.

RDL: How can one tell whether it's a transformation or not? I very seldom feel that I've got an intuitive sense of one thing being a transformation of another. But what I do tend to do is look at anything I hear, including what I say myself, in terms of a plus or minus. So, if someone says anything, makes an affirmation, somewhere or other the affirmation has already implied a negation which is negated. It's a structural inevitability in a binary system that if one set of binary operations is referred to, the other set is virtually there. So, I seldom feel that it does any harm to put to someone the opposite of what's being said, to look at. Not necessarily to say, oh, this is a reaction, the plus is a reaction formation against the minus, or the minus is a reaction formation against the plus. But that there is a plus and minus there, and there is some reason that we have opted for the one or the other. It will always be interesting if someone recoils so much from the negative that they say, oh well that's unthinkable. It can't have been unthinkable because it must have been thought of in order to generate the bifurcation.

AF: So, you're not really implying a value judgement. One thing could be transformed into the other or the other into the one.

RDL: When I try to follow my own emotions around that matrix of jealousy, or what's called jealousy, it all becomes very, very obscure. It's something that Freud never explicitly mentioned. Strindberg is credited with saying that the root of a man's jealousy is the horror and disgust felt at mixing his sperm with another man's.[11] If another man's sperm has got into one's lover's vagina, there is an innate sense of pollution.

I don't know. I must say that I don't like that idea but it is an idea that appeals to a lot of people. In orgies or similar situations, that must be a large part of the attraction. So, it must appeal to some people and have the opposite of an appeal to other people with equal and opposite convictions.

How far would you go in saying, philosophically or epistemologically, that such a psychological question has got an answer, or has a *decidable* answer?

AF: Well, I feel that it becomes a question of ethics and not of psychology.

RDL: Yes, it's always been a question of ethics, anyway. I'm not saying it's not a question of ethics, but without switching from the psychological to the ethical, what would you say about it psychologically? I mean, could we have a formal logic of decidable or undecidable (in principle) types of psychological propositions? It's quite respectable to say that there are some types of propositions which might be very fundamental ones and yet turned out, in principle, using Gödel's proof for instance, to be undecidable.[12]

AF: My guess is that some kind of practical utility function would be involved. Say, two lifestyles may have to be compared as to their costs and benefits. It may not be logically decidable.

RDL: Well, that's not a psychological decision. That's a sort of games-theory, utility decision. I'm talking about trying to decide whether disgust, for instance, is always a reaction formation. Or whether excessive wallowing in shit is in turn a reaction formation against disgust. Such statements are often made, yet by what criteria do you decide whether they are true or false?

Leon Redler: To say that disgust is *always* a reaction formation would be eliminating or denying the possibility of a bifurcation.

RDL: No, that wasn't the proposition. I was wondering whether a particular instance was decidable. I wouldn't even try to answer in general.

LR: Well, sometimes it's knowable. Sometimes one can discover whether disgust is or is not a reactive formation.

RDL: Ah yes. Well, how?

LR: I might have a reaction of disgust or distaste and might not, at the moment of having that reaction, know, but I might subsequently, through whatever happens, come to discover the truth.

RDL: Take a simple thing: For example, I find it disgusting to eat wax from my ears. I wouldn't do that by preference. Especially if it's not fresh. Now, is that a reaction formation, to recoil against that, or not? These reaction formations have to do with effulgences from one's own or other people's bodies. It's either from the ears, the nose, the eyes, the mouth, the genitals, the anus or the skin. For instance, in the height of sexual pleasure, one might love to lick the sweat off of one's partner, right under the armpits, or anywhere! On the other hand, under most circumstances, the idea of licking someone's sweat is disgusting. That's easy to understand because sweat varies enormously with the state that someone is in. I remember when I was in analysis with Rycroft, I was married to my first wife, Anne. We had four children, and a fifth child, Adrian, was born just around that time. I told him that I didn't find it disgusting to have sexual intercourse with my wife when she was menstruating, especially as it was by far the safest time. Rycroft didn't insist, but he put it to me that he found this very unusual and he said maybe I was denying a more basic sense of disgust, or at least a sort of primitive sense of segregation.

AF: When I was in analysis in Toronto, it came up that, after ejaculation, I don't lose my erection. My analyst said, "You're lying."

RDL: Well, that's a good example of a rather simple-minded psychoanalytic construction. I wouldn't even call it an interpretation. It's just a construction on the situation that you are denying that you've come. Well, how can that be decided? And that's just a particular instance. If you caved in and agreed with him, it might only mean that you had submitted to power, to hypnosis. If you kept your end up, so to speak, and refused to buckle down, it might just mean that you were resistant. I would bet, for instance, not very much because it's obviously hedged in different ways, that if we did a survey of Americans of voting age, we would find that more Democrats than Republicans had looked at their own assholes in the mirror. Wouldn't you think so?

LR: What makes you say that?

RDL: Well, there are some people who have seen their own assholes and some people who haven't. Some people have never looked at their own behinds, never used a mirror to look.

AF: What's the construct you're using to link up political affiliation with asshole-gazing?

RDL: I think it's a natural curiosity to look at one's own body and to look at every part of one's body at least once. So, I would place a construction on that: someone who hasn't done so is inhibited. Their relationship to the object around which they are inhibited will be distorted in different ways. Things to do with shit and assholes are liable to be projected, therefore, more in people who have never looked at their own assholes or even looked at their own shit. I wouldn't say handling it is necessary, or tasting it, but at least seeing one's own shit, actually looking at the composition of what comes out of one... I would think that people who can't do that are more liable to develop ultra-right politically because their political fantasy would be to some extent a biased, projected, anal ideology, in the absence of direct access to their own anus. It's possible that

Democrats are not as tarnished by the process as Republicans. Wouldn't you think there must be that sort of correlation?

AF: This is reminiscent of the psychohistorians, such as Lloyd deMause.

LR: Why do you think someone who is ultra-left might not have the same number going?

RDL: I think anyone who is ultra is liable to have the same number going. I would have to generalise by saying that I think people who don't have a reflective relationship with their own shit are more liable to find their own shit coming at them from the external world. They are living in a world in which they've got to defend themselves from shit coming at them.

All of this is a very complex system of construction, so if you don't agree with it, it must sound desperately arrogant and completely scientifically arbitrary. But it's not a single individual quirk. I mean, if one puts an idea like that out in a sufficiently coherent way, millions of people will immediately say, "Aha! Yes absolutely. I completely agree with that. You are just voicing another nuance of the way we think already, and you're so right!" Others, who don't agree with it, find it a very offensive argument, I mean deeply offensive, uncivilised even.

AF: Lloyd deMause has his theory that the first generation of unswaddled babies were the ones who grew up to lead the fight of the American Revolution.[13] That's a similar construction, not perhaps as complicated as yours, but it's unprovable. All the same, some people say, "Aha, that's right!" and others, "That's crazy!"

LYING

AF: For the practitioner of brief therapy, anything goes: they feign and lie, they cheat right and left, bamboozling the people they work with. I wonder if lying can be used to raise hope or if lying can be deployed positively. I suspect brief therapy may *have* to be *brief* (three to five sessions), because you can't lie *and* sustain a relationship for any length of time. If you lie, you better finish the relationship quickly.

RDL: I don't know whether that's true but it's an interesting thought. Aren't there chronic lies? Lies that people keep up for a lifetime?

LR: Aren't there relationships that are very much founded on deceit? You might say that it's not a *real* relationship, that it's a sham, but...

AF: Would this be true: lying doesn't make sense between friends? Lying only makes sense between enemies.

RDL: Is that true though?

AF: Well, I'm wondering. I'm putting that forward as a hypothesis. Why would you lie to a friend?

RDL: Well, suppose someone is a friend but has got a very weak spot, something that matters far too much to him or her for their own good, but they're not going to get out of it right away, and they put one of those all or nothing questions to you, say, "Am I any good at it?" or "Am I an attractive woman/man?"
I was with Alan Watts and his wife once, who had just crawled out of a sanatorium outside Paris, having had a hypoglycemic crisis and was expected to have another one.[14] She hadn't been cured and she looked absolutely awful just then. Anyway, we

got into one of those very sort-of frank discussions in which I said to her that her whole trouble was that she had the image of herself as an attractive woman. If she just gave that up, she wouldn't have any more problems. This had quite a lot of repercussions, as I gathered from Alan later. He brought it up *years* later. I don't think I should have done that! Imagine a similar situation where you are asked a question, the real answer to which would cause a great deal of pain to the person who heard the truth. The clear and straightforward truth might not be absolutely necessary to tell. In other words, even a slight distortion of the truth, sufficient to call it a lie, might obviate the pain. The truth or the lie might not contain any particular enlightenment about anything.

AF: Is one justified in generating hope, even at the cost of having to falsify certain information? Can *false* hope be healing?

RDL: All that I was saying was in response to your saying that lying doesn't arise between friends. I think it arises very much between people who love each other deeply. When it comes to severe illness or death, a spouse might feel, out of love, that he or she ought not to tell them that they are dying.

AF: My guess is that if a long-term relationship were based on deceit, it would be two people living together like enemies. Their life-long relationship would be based on animosity.

RDL: It might also be based on a sort of love. Reading the life and times in the nineteenth century, say, take an imaginary paradigmatic Victorian marriage from the pages of the *Goncourt Journal*, which was read by and written about Gustave Flaubert, Émile Zola, Ivan Turgenev, the historian Hippolyte Taine and many others, and you get this picture of a man and his wife: he'll go to brothels but he doesn't want his wife to know *because* he loves her. At least that's the rhetoric. And not just because of the pain that would arise between them but because he doesn't want to hurt her. He doesn't want her to know, whereas if a man doesn't give a fuck about his wife, or hates her, he'll rub her nose in it. The truth is used cruelly in order to hurt. Sometimes, something is actually done in order for it to be heard about, in order to create a painful truth. In other words, a man will have a mistress in order to create a fact which, being true, will hurt his wife and humiliate her and subject her to all sorts of social degradation. The truth can be used in a foul way. Whereas a lie, though it leads to the question of whether *ultimately* all lies are absolutely wrong, nevertheless can be told in the opposite way, to avoid hurting somebody. I can imagine such secrets must sometimes go right to the grave when a lifetime of deceit has gone into maintaining an appearance which has been kept up, which has given pleasure and security and was never meant to be broken.

AF: Lying doesn't seem to be identified as a sin in the Bible.

LR: When does it first come up? Isn't it with Adam and Eve? Isn't there an original lie there? Don't they initially deny hearing God calling them?

RDL: Was it Jacob and Esau?

LR: Yes, that's right.

RDL: That was a major lie.

If one's being tortured and one has to lie to save one's friends, all the sorts of people who would say they're on the side of truth would most certainly say they're on the side of lying. There must be something wrong with the argument "Tell the truth, whether it betrays your friends or not, and you've got no problem: just adhere to the truth." The truth is a metaphor. It's Truth with a capital T, and it doesn't absolutely refer to printing an accurate railway timetable or to saying where someone is at some time. I mean, you can say the truth of the relationships between two people might entail lying.

LR: This came up recently with me and one of my kids, Hannah. We got into talking about lying and I said that I really felt that I, for myself, wanted to tell the truth and not to lie whenever possible, and hoped she felt the same way. Truth-telling seems to be the right action and yet it seems very important to be able to lie. There are certainly times when it is necessary to lie in order to save a life: mine or someone else's.

AF: So, there must be some higher organising principle than the one governing whether to lie or not.

RDL: Terribly tricky.

LR: Well, I would say "Do no one harm!" seems to be of a higher moral and spiritual principle than "Do not lie!" The right action might involve lying.

RDL: That's an important point. The early Christians were apparently very occupied with this problem. They developed the theory of equivocation.[15] Suppose that you, a member of a condemned religious sect, were stopped in the street by a Roman security guard: "Where are you going? Are you going to a religious meeting?" Well, if you're a slave, you can say, "I am going to the house of my lord," which means "I'm going to the house of my master slaveholder" or "I'm going to a religious meeting/church." This was classified as "equivocation", *not* lying.

Why bother with equivocation, a sort of nicety of conscience? Why not just be straight and admit the issue in full force? I haven't fully confronted that. For a number of years, I thought lying was just an expedient, then I began to feel that to lie was a more serious spiritual error, and now I am faced with complicated situations that do not allow these simple separations.

AF: I want to bring up the question of self-deception. I think it's crazy to lie to oneself, and therefore it's crazy to lie to anyone who one considers very close to oneself. The closer someone is to me, the crazier it would be for me to lie to them. The further away someone is from me, the more it may make sense to lie on occasion.

RDL: I think it's a more important question to ask who lies to whom. I mean, if oneself is who one takes oneself to be, it doesn't really matter terribly much whether one lies to oneself, because oneself has got one's number.

AF: But I may have internalised enemies.

RDL: You *can't* lie to yourself! I mean, *yourself* is that from which the data comes out of to supply you with the information for the construction of the lie. There is absolutely no point in lying to oneself.

LR: You seem to be saying that you can't lie to yourself, not just that it's pointless.

RDL: Oh, you *can* lie to yourself, but you're wasting your time. My self has supplied me with the data with which I then may try to lie to it. But it already knows everything that I'm trying to censor. It's like a censor getting a book from an author, censoring the book and returning it, in fact telling the author that they haven't written this or that. The author has provided all the sentences the censor is erasing, so they can erase it as much as they like, but why convince the author that they never wrote what got censored? It's a bad thing for me to lie to myself. The question is whether I can trust myself not to lie to me. Polonius, in *Hamlet*, gives the most well-known advice: "To thine own self be true!"

AF: I wonder how different that is from "Know thyself!"[16]

RDL: What do the words "know" and "true" mean? I mean, what is the relationship of truth? What is the ontologically true relationship, as *adequatio*, between *intellectu* and *in rei*?[17] We're not even talking about between *intellectu* and *in rei*, we're talking existentially between oneself and oneself. So we have to state, you might say, the comparative morphology of what a true relationship is. Heidegger argued that we should abandon worrying about an *adequatio* and thing of truth, imagine it, intuit it more as an unveiling, a revealing. There are many metaphors that express this in terms of two opposing concepts, like illusion and reality or the counterfeit and the genuine. This is played upon a great deal in East Indian metaphysics: we see this tinsel and we take it to be silver. I suppose this is an illusion of construction. What we see is just what we see but we place our own construction on it. We take it to be different from what it is.

CHANGE

AF: I'd like to talk about the all-pervasive problem of working with people in a therapeutic situation, using well-articulated theories or techniques. Working on the west coast of North America, there is certainly a proliferation of well-articulated techniques and theories. More and more, I suspect that such approaches just postpone the moment of truth when a person could encounter their true self. A lot of pseudo-change occurs in therapy as somebody sorts out what the technique or theory of the moment is and develops a new false self from an old false self, creating the *illusion* of change. To put it in hypnotic terms, it's as if there is a change of programmer but there is no awakening. Maybe the only way to de-hypnotise people is by refusing to be their new hypnotist.

RDL: There is no way one person can wake up someone else, as far as I know. There is a sense in which, if you are asleep, I can give you a nudge, call your name, and I can wake you up. Any alarm clock can wake anyone up. The sleep/waking situation, however, is only an analogy. There is a sleep and a waking state, and there is a certain state of waking consciousness that we say is, in some way, akin to sleep, from which we hope you will wake up. We revert to that analogy because we haven't got a primary way of talking about the thing in itself. Now, I think, the analogy breaks down all over the place, and very quickly, when we think there might be professional, skilful, scientific or intuitive ways and means in which we can substitute the role of the alarm clock, expecting a paradoxical behaviour prescription or an interpretation to wake you up.

AF: A better analogy, then, is that, if one just refrains from feeding new dreams, the person *may* wake up by themselves.

RDL: Yeah, if someone is in a state of carbon monoxide poisoning, they may or may not come out of it, but it would certainly help to turn off the gas and provide some oxygen to breathe. But there are no guarantees. Obviously, you stop, as far as possible, dishing out the poison, and provide a psychologically non-toxic environment that is not facilitating them going to sleep. In the Christian tradition, it's a matter of grace, and God alone effects that conversion. You can't open the door from this side of it. You can knock. It's only opened from the other side. No secular power, temporal power, or individual psyches, the therapist's or the patient's, can open that door.

AF: So, do you feel that choosing gestalt therapy, transactional analysis or psychoanalysis is beside the point because it doesn't really matter what one engages in, either plus or minus?[18]

RDL: It of course depends on the spirit in which it's conducted. I mean, the spirit in which it's conducted really does critically affect any procedure, and I think it is the main determining factor. The most superb spiritual disciplines are out in the marketplace, from prayer, to mantras, to you name it! A lot of people, whom I suppose the three of us would regard as wise, have agreed that it's a good thing for people to occupy their time doing things. Whether it's cobblering or meditating, it's neither plus nor minus *what* you do, as long as you don't do harm. Pretty well everyone has said: "Don't do harm intentionally." A lot of people have also said: "It's a good thing to keep at it and keep on trying, even if only to realise that you won't get anywhere entirely by your own efforts." We're told to pray, we're told even to beseech, we're told to put our best foot forward and do what we can, even though at the same time, we're told that no amount of good works, which I suppose includes psychotherapy, can force open access to what one is hoping to get at. The door can't be forced from this side of it. We can make a clamour on this side of it, we have even been told to knock and, as it is said, "it shall be opened unto you."[19] Certainly, a lot of people have felt that they asked until they were blue in the face and there was no answer. The answer very likely doesn't come in the form that the question has been asked. Since there is some reformation necessary to the state of mind that asked the question, one can't really expect an answer on one's own terms.

AF: Alexis Carrel, a Nobel Prize-winning doctor, went to Lourdes to check out what was really happening there. He concluded that people do get healed, and what he felt was the effective ingredient was the *quality* of the prayer. The prayer had to be non-specific, not asking, "Please Lord, heal my knee!" or "let me walk again!" What worked was offering yourself up to God's mercy, so to speak. As he put it, the quality of the prayer must be a state of love and submission to God, not a selfish desire for recovery.[20]

RDL: Here we come to one of those apparent paradoxes.

AF: The treasure at the bottom of the deep well can be yours, as long as you don't think of a white monkey while you are descending.

RDL: Well, the stereotype of the pilgrim to Lourdes is the cripple or the desperately miserable ill person who is going there to beseech God to mercifully relieve them of their physical affliction. Yet, if they ask for that, they won't get it. Perhaps, carried away by the spirit of the place, paradoxically, one can forget that what one has come about is one's own misery. You can't even say "Thy will be done!" because it's a bit impertinent, really! "Thy will" is, obviously, being done. All you can do is thank God in jubilation, without any protest for His will being done, absolutely not asking for anything, just rejoicing in His will being done. Obviously, the state I'm in is by "Thy will," no one else's, so, what am I praying about!? At that point, someone might get up and walk!

AF: During an LSD session, there was a point at which I was heading toward something like a death experience. As long as even a tiny part of my mind was wishing and anticipating – "Oh, good, I'm going to die now!" – the experience eluded me, it just fizzled out, went away, never happened. On a few occasions, I got really scared that maybe I overdosed, that maybe this is it, maybe something's going wrong, and for a moment I wasn't gleeful but scared about death approaching. *Then* it happened, with me no longer in control, but swept away.

RDL: I've always found it difficult to pray for any change in myself or in my own life because of a sense of impertinence. This is a very deep paradox: "Thy will be done on earth as it is in heaven." The English form, at any rate, seems to imply that His will isn't being done on earth, otherwise why pray that it be done? This is a statement that it is being done in heaven. No doubt heaven is where it's being done. If it's being done, it's no doubt in heaven.

AF: It's as if from Houston, Texas, say, we send some robots out to a different planet. For them, Houston, Texas would be in heaven, right? And then, these robots could be praying for good reception of radio signals so as to carry out accurately what is dictated to them from heaven.

LR: One prays to learn and *know* "Thy will."

RDL: We are also told that the Kingdom of Heaven is within us. It's not in Houston, Texas.

AF: Well, there may be noise and poor signal detection from the headquarters *within* us.

RDL: We're cut off, we're cursed, we're expelled or we're excluded from our own deepest access to the Kingdom of Heaven which we find within us. All right, presumably there is no real peace from a spiritual point of view if that state of accursedness continues. We can expect biological, social, emotional, psychological and mental repercussions at all levels of our accursed selves. It seems to be a very common fantasy that professionals, in all the therapies that are proliferating today, can quickly get at this state we are in and blast us out of it and have the power to blow us out of this damned state. They go on about how they abreact them, gestalt them and primal them.[21] In other words, have it out, get into it, get the roots up, etc., etc. We don't see going around the world are sort of elite primal-therapy saints, shining lights all over the place. Look at Janov, a miserable paranoid creature who thinks of nothing else but how he's been ripped off, not appreciated, and misunderstood and ripped off again. He'll fly a thousand miles to go to a country where he thinks his books are being published without him getting his fair quota of royalties in order to try and ferret it out.

AF: Are there risks involved in being a healer or a therapist?

RDL: There certainly are risks involved but I don't know whether it's more hazardous than many other activities.

AF: There is a Hungarian shaman legend, according to which every time a shaman does a genuine healing, a member of their family dies. So they don't do very many.

RDL: I think there is a cost like that in all human activity. I don't think it's quite right to compare the white Western therapist with a shaman. There are many different sorts of shamans. Joan Halifax's latest book is quite useful in that respect.[22] It shows one shaman, one who is typical of many others, who reminds me of Freddie Ayer, the Oxford analytic professor of philosophy: very intellectual. Shamans do different sorts of things. Some shamans specialise in releasing evil spirits. I know such a shaman. He is a minister who is an exorcist's exorcist. His church is nearby. He thinks that what you do, what happens in an exorcism of an evil spirit, is that you actually release it from prison or from its playground and force out of someone an evil spirit. That doesn't dispose of the evil spirit, it stays around in this actual same space looking for someone else to get into. This, of course, could be the exorcist, or anyone close to them: close, not in space-time, but in their psychosphere. There it becomes a dangerous, loose creature who is out to do the next person in.

AF: You don't think, then, that there is a great danger to you when working with someone? That something that's going on with them could infect you or poison you?

RDL: I have had that fantasy or feeling or experience. A number of times, I certainly felt it in those terms. Some people are definitely dangerous. I mean dangerous because what they've got in them is liable to get into oneself or someone close to one. On one occasion, my wife, Jutta, started to act towards me exactly in the character and with the intonation of a woman patient of mine who had recently got, you might say, better. Fortunately, it didn't stick.

AF: Did Jutta know the woman?

RDL: No, no, she didn't. That was the remarkable thing. One possibility of transmission was through me, including through subtle kinesics and paralinguistics of a basic dynamic gestalt of someone else. It seemed to evaporate within just a few minutes. I've come to allow for the existence of an ESP domain, however it's characterised. There is some very deep connection between our individual psyches. Jutta has been very apprehensive about me getting involved in any stuff to do with exorcism. She'd be happier if I didn't even go along to observe one of this minister's exorcisms. He is about to do one and invited me. He's been at me for years to come along when he does it and I've kept away from it. A South African woman will be exorcised, who is being ruined by a curse that was put on her by a Black African witchdoctor woman.

AF: Are you going to go?

RDL: Yeah, I am going to go to it. It will be done in church with his full regalia on, of course.

AF: About four years ago, you said once you were really interested in hypnosis and maybe you would do more work in it.

RDL: Yes, I haven't done anything about that yet. I haven't developed anything at all.

LR: Is that a particularly strong interest of yours that is lying low for the while?

RDL: No, but I've done a certain amount of hypnosis for several years and then gave it up. I've never got back into it. It's a very

interesting field, very open for grabs. It's quite easy to hypnotise someone and put them through numbers which only an
accomplished yogi could go through. Under hypnosis, you can
put someone through the extremes, really, of any routine that
accomplished people go through. If we hypnotised you, and
told you that this metronome is beating at 60 beats a minute,
then slowed down the metronome, your heartbeat would slow
down. You would believe it was beating at 60 per minute when
in fact it was beating at 30. Your speech would slow down too.
Did you ever see a documentary film that shows Osmond doing just exactly that?[23] The woman used in that experiment
actually ended up in the mental hospital afterwards. The subject was hypnotised and she'd been told the metronome was
beating 60 ticks per minute. The tick-tock slowed down, and
as it slowed down, her words become slower, slower… just
like a record. Her movements slowed down. Eventually, it
stopped and she became motionless for about two minutes
until the tick started again, and then her movement started up.
Then it got faster and she became clinically manic. Not only
did her words and movements become faster but, of course,
her associations became faster, and the pitch of her voice also
became higher. It is not immediately obvious why the pitch
should vary like that.

SHAMANISM, HEALING AND R.D. LAING. *By Francis Huxley**

Times do change. Fancy being asked to speak on the subject of shamanism, healing, and R. D. Laing – of Laing, who was not a shaman but a psychiatrist, and here, under the auspices of what he took to be the House of Rimmon, the temple of anti-psychiatry, where he figured as the anti-psychiatrist in person.[1] I might not have so readily agreed to this, had not Laing once told me that, when invited to meet the Pope, he refused because, he said, he'd never live it down if he did. But now that he'd missed the chance, he hardly knew how to live that down either.

I am, as our chairman has told you, a social anthropologist, and before I met Laing, I had the chance to live with a Brazilian tribe and learn about shamans and cannibalism, among other things: to have worked in an overcrowded Canadian mental hospital, to have taken an ethnopsychiatric look at vaudoun (voodoo) in Haiti, to have been intimate with a Brazilian practitioner who, though he came out of a possession cult, was shamanising as a solo act, etc. etc. etc., as Laing was wont to say.

Such are my credentials for speaking as I do, and as they were for Laing when he invited me to join the Philadelphia Association. They also give me reason to ask why shamanism should be relevant when speaking of Laing, sexy word though it is these days. For Laing was not a shaman. It wasn't his style. He didn't beat drums, shake rattles, brandish crystals, blow tobacco smoke on his clients or make a show of sucking out the nasties. He didn't invoke his guiding spirit with songs and then fall into epileptoid fits, nor did he eat burning coals, slit his belly open, ventriloquise, or get into sorcery or divination. He prescribed no remedies, did no conjuring tricks and did not hurl magic darts on the sly.

Nor was he a possession priest of a cult such as vaudoun, candomble, makumba, umbanda or spiritismo. These are Haitian and Brazilian forms of African possession cults, and their initiates go all the way from being conventionally normal to unconventionally abnormal, sometimes with a vengeance. I found much of interest in these cults, such as their method of diagnosing an illness in terms of their client's daimon, their native character, rather than in those typifying the disorder, per se. They do this by discerning which of a pantheon of Loa, of gods and spirits, is the ruling spirit of their clients. By initiating them into the mysteries of possession by that particular Loa, they manage to expel the others that have arbitrarily installed themselves in their clients' psychic economy, and so take over the direction of their lives.

The effectiveness of this highly ritualised approach may be gauged by what happened when a Haitian troupe put on vaudoun ceremonies in France, some forty years ago. Quite a few spectators were then possessed by the relevant Loa of the ritual moment even though the audience was entirely unfamiliar with such goings-on. (Maya Deren, in *The Divine Horsemen*, reports a more complex experience of this kind that happened to herself.) A sociologist who had witnessed the affair discovered that those possessed had all been under some form of therapeutic treatment, and that after their possession, they felt so much saner that, for a year, none of them had found cause to return to medical forms of relief.

But Laing was not a possession priest any more than he was a shaman. Could you call him a Nabi? Nabi is the Hebrew word the Bible translates as prophet (which Laing certainly was, in his own way), those who speak vehemently in God's name, calling for repentance, admonishing the ungodly and being consulted by kings about politics. They also heal: Elisha, for example, cured Naaman the Syrian of leprosy, who then declared he believed there was no God except that of Israel, and asked forgiveness if he had to accompany his king into the House of Rimmon and bow there. (Go in peace, Elisha told him.) Nabis of this kind are now defunct in Israel, though according to Margaret Field, in *Search for Security*, they flourish in Ghana as possession priests, diviners, magicians, healers and exorcists.[2]

But are such latter-day Nabis, Nabis proper? For that matter, what distinguishes them from shamans? Mircea Eliade, when discussing shamanism, defined the vocation as the ability to keep self-witness when taken by a fit of inspiration, and set it apart from possession cults in which self-witness is lost.[3] There are so many exceptions to this rule in both camps, however, as to make it nugatory. Even in the heartland of shamanism proper, most shamans are possessed by their spirits – mounted by them, Haitians would say – before being able to ride them: while in vaudoun the final stage of initiation, which authorises a servitor to set up a temple and control its activities, is known as *"la prise des yeux"*, the taking hold of the eyes. This is a state in which, for all the nearly intolerable turmoil occasioned by a full inspirational upsurge, the privileged victims are able to retain self-witness. Such being the case, it is best to recast the question in terms of the inspirational fit and the different theatres of action in which it displays itself, the difficulty of retaining self-witness being the same whatever the style adopted.

There is yet one mark by which a Nabi proper may be distinguished from one half-made or merely pretending, as there is with a shaman or a possession priest. This being what, in the Bible, is called the discernment of spirits – an instant recognition of what afflicts a client, together with the ability to get to the heart of the matter on the spur of the moment. True, the gift is not restricted to them, as I hardly need remind you: I have known a doctor who could diagnose at twenty paces, as well as a philosopher, a painter, a novelist, a psychotherapist or two of various persuasions, a garage mechanic, a priest and of course Laing himself, who could do as much. All the same, it is an arduous task to perfect this gift, for though it is native to us all, it is commonly repressed – with some reason, for it goes to that place where the sense of one's self is permeated by the sense of others, often to one's confusion.

What then is the nature of self-witness? I take it that S.T. Coleridge was speaking to this point when he said that the organs of spiritual sense were consubstantial with their objects – a profound remark from a man who evidently knew as much by direct experience.[4] And so it was with Coventry Patmore when he declared love to be "that marvellous state in which each of two persons in distinct bodies perceives sensibly all that the other feels in regard to him or herself, although their feelings are of the most opposite characteristics."[5] One cannot say as much, unfortunately, for Lucien Levy-Bruhl, whose writings on mystical participation suffer accordingly or, for that matter, for modern physicists who hold, without even appealing to Werner Heisenberg, that if two particles are identical in their behaviour, they may safely be counted as one.[6]

As much to the point is the sense of being what one perceives during nightmares. I mention nightmare for its close association with possession states, as the literature on the subject makes clear, while folklore records the saving grace of such an experience by advising the sufferer to take a nightmare by its toe, when it will transform into a voluptuous moment. This, along with what Coleridge and Patmore have declared, tells us that the two-fold sense of consubstantial mutuality is also the breeding ground of personifications, and raises the problem of how to deal with them when they get out of hand.

Here then is what I take to be the actual subject I have been asked to speak upon today. A subject whose natural focus is an I–Thou moment – this being when a two-fold sense meets another two-fold sense – whose energetics are well characterised in Jacob Boehme's words "the being of beings is a wrestling power".[7]

Every shaman I have met, and every member of a possession cult, would agree that such is the case, as of course Laing would have, along with many another, whatever their vocation. For shamanism is a vocation – the utmost of vocations – in that its practitioners are called to it much as they might wish to avoid that laborious, painful and alienating destiny. How should it not be, when they first hear its voice in a nightmare, into which they again fall, should they cease to shamanise, as happened to Jonah – Jonah the scapegoat? Or, if you prefer, the wounded healer.

I take it, meanwhile, that the awakening of the two-fold sense to its own existence is part and parcel of initiation in general. An event that is usually staged at puberty as a horror story accompanied by painful moments of every kind, with a view to awaken the young to their place in the scheme of things. However, quite a number of people wake up to this, their self-witness, at a much earlier age. Eileen Garret, who had once been Arthur Conan Doyle's trance-medium, told me that she had woken up in this fashion when, at the age of four, she was harshly reprimanded by her parents for telling them of an event she thought natural, but which they regarded as supernaturally disrespectful even to mention. Mid-life crises may also provide the occasion for such awakenings.

What has been called the shamanic illness usually strikes around puberty, but by no means always, and takes much the same form whatever the diagnosis, according to Western custom. Epilepsy was, for a time, a favourite diagnosis, soon to be followed by arctic hysteria, which under other names was recognised by tribal peoples whose women-folk were especially prone to it – brought on by those long sunless winters, and blizzards in which, the Inuit say, one can hear the spirits of the dead howling their recriminations. Knud Rasmussen, that best of past ethnographers, tells of how they countered this dismal affect when he and a party of Inuit were caught in just such a blizzard. After slogging through it for terrible hours, they found shelter in the ruins of a summer dwelling. Rasmussen collapsed behind a wall, but not so his companions – to his amazed vexation, they set about making themselves snug. They talked, they laughed and they sang. "How can you be singing after all we've gone through?" he at last inquired. "Ah," said one of them, "if we weren't happy, we would die."[8] This was also Laing's view: he not only extolled the virtues of conviviality but made a point of setting it in motion by getting people to sing Noel Coward songs, or Victorian ones, such as "O for the Wings of a Dove" or "The Lost Chord", while accompanying them on the piano. Though I admit there were other times when he was in such an unconvivial mood, his companions were afflicted with hesitation and gloom. He rather enjoyed such moments, I suspect, for the insights they gave him into what happens to a group when deprived of an agenda. A practice in which W. R. Bion excelled by remaining steadfastly unconvivial whatever the mood of his group.

Then there's tropical hysteria – that is, latah – for which quite another explanation must be found. There are the effects of traumatic shock, as when an Inuit had his kayak overturned by an enraged walrus that tusked him through the lungs. His companions saw him to the shore of ice, built him an igloo and left him there for days without dressing his wounds, lighting an oil lamp, or providing him with food. And that's how he became an angekok, a shaman. And then there are shamans that have been diagnosed as schizothymic, schizophrenic, idiopathic-paranoiac, etc. etc., who have recovered some if not all of their senses by undergoing the classical shamanic experience of being dismembered, tormented and remade with iron bones or rock-crystals stolen from the sky, with one, two, even seven bones left over, which represent new and special powers.

Powers which, alas, have to be paid for indirectly with the life of one of the shaman's immediate family. (Such things happen closer to home: see Laing's writings on the family.)

Having sketched this outline of what it is to be a shaman, I may now bring in R.D. Laing on his own count. For though he was a psychiatrist and not a shaman, I must now so far contradict myself as to hold that he yet had a shamanic temperament. I don't suppose this to be all that different from the creative temperament, whether it be artistic or scientific. A notable instance of this last being Nikola Tesla, the ipsissimus of electricity – or psychological, as exemplified by C.G. Jung in self, both of whom have left accounts of their awakening to its existence. I don't know when Laing woke up in like vein, fairly early I suppose. I never heard, though I do know under whose patronage he may be said to have done so, for he told me. He had just come back from Iona, and paid me an unexpected visit. I gave him a drink. He stood with an elbow on the mantelpiece and, after a companionable silence, told me he was, as it were, a reincarnation of St Odran, whose legend he started to tell me. He did so with such stumbles and rollings-up of the eyes, I thought to save him the trouble of switching on his memory by looking into the top of his head. "But I've just come across the story myself," I broke in, found the book, *Ten Thousand Saints: A Study of Irish and European Origins* by Hubert Butler, turned to the page and read the précis of the legend aloud:

St Odran was a famous saint of Iona. It is said that St Columba, finding that demons were infesting a site [where he wished to build a chapel – St Odran's chapel, it is now called], discovered that only by burying a holy man alive could they be exorcised. St Odran volunteered but after three days, Columba decided to dig him up again for news of Heaven. St. Odran, on being uncovered, instead of giving suitable information said, "There is no wonder in Death, and Hell is not as it is reported." Thereupon Columba cried out furiously: "Earth, earth upon the mouth of Odran that he may blab no more!" And he was covered up again.[9]

Laing heard me out with an approving smile, which I thought friendly of him, and then said that Odran must have been a priest of the Irish goddess before his conversion to Christianity, by which he had hoped to escape her attentions. (She is the Morrigan, mother of all, demons included, and the vengeant queen of love in death.) There was no need for me to do more than smile in my turn, though not without a sigh.

Earth, earth, upon the mouth of Laing that he should blab no more about there being no wonder in psychiatry, and that schizophrenia is not as it is reported. But I only learnt the context of this revelation at his funeral, when the Reverend Donald Macdonald mounted the pulpit to give the oration. He told of Laing's visit to Iona, their meeting, their hot-tempered quarrelling over religious matters, and the fight they got into before Laing submitted himself to the authority of the Church of Scotland. In proof of which he took a blood-stained prayer book from his pocket, and held it above his head. The gesture was as eloquent as the words the "duke of dark corners" spoke to the miserable Claudio in Shakespeare's *Measure for Measure*:

Be absolute for death – death or life
Shall thereby be the sweeter

Words I am sure Laing would have approved of when he came to require this unconditionality of himself. He was then trusting his inspiration without second thought, as he had not quite been doing when it had been his wont to say "I don't even trust my own judgement unless I have to."

The being of beings is indeed a wrestling power, and in meeting it, Laing had the advantage of being something of a Glaswegian brawler. How he liked fighting and putting himself to physical test, if it was only playing rugby when he was young. This in spite of all his piano teacher said against it, for sure enough someone stepped on his hand and broke some bones. Not ruinously (for he was as deft in playing nightclub music as that of Bach, where I most admired his talent) but enough to scotch any idea that he could make a career of it.

Instead, he took to psychiatry as a profession, and as his shamanic temperament no doubt played a part in this choice, a brief word about its nature is due. He had no quarrel with his father, who was a professional singer, but with his mother, he once told me. Was she perhaps, he wondered, Jewish? That would explain why, when he was a child, she kept his cup, saucer, plate and cutlery apart, with repeated injunctions to his father not to touch. (But touch he would on occasion, with a mocking smile.) She also insisted on giving him his bath till he was of an age to lock the door against her, and for all her hammerings, kicks and screams of rage, she had to own defeat. Much later, he heard from someone in the family that she had made a doll in his name and was sticking pins in it. On his next visit, he asked her about that. A short silence, and then "We don't talk about such things," she replied.

And there was that further time, quite early on, when his father gave her a present on her birthday. Never before had he known his father to give her anything on any occasion, but there it was, a small box neatly wrapped, tied with a ribbon. She looked at it for a while, then slowly unknotted the ribbon, unwrapped the paper, took the lid off, removed a layer of cotton wool, and what should she see but the clippings of ten fingernails and ten toenails in orderly array. Not a word said she, not a glance she gave to her husband, but rose from her chair and left the room, leaving an ominous silence behind her.

I heard this story years after I had ventured to give him a Christmas present. He showed me into his study, which I hadn't seen before and was much impressed by the dark green of its walls, in whose shade the most lonely could feel at home with the Alone, even in company. Laing unwrapped the small bronze Buddha hand that I had brought. He was then practising meditation, and when it lay open to his gaze, I became acutely aware of the pugnacious wings of his nose and the scorn-lines that ran down from them. Then, after a moment's thought, he got up from his chair, opened a cupboard, reached in and came out with a sword stick, which he negligently handed to me.

It was a dreadful object, ugly, heavy, and unwieldy both as a stick and a sword. The handle was perfunctory and the wood of the scabbard-stick worm-holed to the breaking point. A real old-time blackguard's weapon it was, and I could just see him as a young man buying it in a Glasgow junk shop and keeping it until the telling moment arrived to rid himself of it at another's expense. As I accepted this dubious comment on myself, delivered as it was in the confines of his dark green room, I began to wonder what he thought I had thought I was doing in giving him a present.

He told me as much twenty years later, when I came with another gift for his last child, then just born. Again, he bridled with distaste, remembering how our mutual friend Joan Westcott, an anthropologist who for a time had been his secretary, had once given him a crucifix made of rifle bullets with a tin Jesus soldered to it, First World War vintage. It wasn't that he didn't appreciate the object, for it was on his mantelpiece for years, but that Joan, noticing his discomfort, lectured him on the anthropology of the gift, of how it created a web of social relationships by putting the recipient under an obligation to give something back. "An obligation," he repeated with horror.

To give is indeed a two-faced operation, for the same word does duty, in its various cognates, for giving, having, receiving and taking. While in German, *das Gift* means poison. It may rightly stand, therefore, as epitomising the double bind, such as makes a divided self of its victim. Laing got the term from Gregory Bateson, who had arrived at it after lengthily wrestling with a ceremony of role reversal, Naven by name, practised by a tribe in New Guinea, a knotty problem involving several forms of two-fold sense. Meanwhile, Laing got the idea of a knot from a Sufi poem, and his book of *Knots* shows him at his minimalist best, though it does not include the most heart-rending of these sickest of jokes. This, which in his later years I often heard him repeat with heroic despair, represents – so Jutta Laing has told me – an interchange he had with his mother at an early age. It goes like this:

Do you love me?
Yes.
Do you believe me?
Yes.
How can you love me if you believe me?

I am sorry to say that *The Lies of Love*, his last book, is still unpublished. For those who have read it tell me they were much engaged by its disturbing reports of similar interchanges. Laing indeed detested lies above all things and would go out of his way to demolish liars. Nor did he ever forget his bafflement when a couple came to see him with such contradictory and yet persuasive stories that he was unable to determine which of the two was lying about what, such a mare's nest had they made for themselves to lie in together.

There were also times when Laing found himself in yet deeper and darker waters, which involved not just double binds – spells, an anthropologist might well call them – but curses. One instance, of which he published a brief account, had to do with a woman who cursed her son to the seventh generation so successfully that four generations later, his sole descendant realised he would also be the last. He had made every effort to free himself from his fate but, he said, it was like one of those Russian dolls that had smaller ones inside, all of which he could deal with, but the innermost – entirely beyond appeal – was the mother still mouthing her implacable curse.

I have known of curses being removed by vaudouists, as long as the curser was still alive, but not when the curse had renewed itself over successive generations. A Tibetan exorcist might, from the little I know of such practitioners, have done better, though the wrestling power involved is beyond my comprehension, and by all accounts takes so much out of an exorcist that such men usually die in their thirties. Laing's nearest approach to such a feat that I know of concerned one of the first, most chronic inhabitants of a Philadelphia Association household, David by name, who had just returned from hospital in a high state of mania. Laing gave him what I once heard him call his undivided attention ("No thanks" was Andrew Feldmár's response when offered it, ha-ha, as a birthday present.) He did this silently and without looking at him, so well that David soon fell silent. Laing then told the others present what he had done, whereupon David took flight again. Laing once more set himself to attend, again David fell silent. What he had done, he later told me, was to take David's frenzy and contain it in himself. But the effect on him was so great that, when he left, soon after, to drive himself home, Laing collapsed in the car from the strain. David, meanwhile, was back in high-speed mania.

This same David spoke a rapid and advanced form of schizophrenese which, exhausting though it was to attend to, Laing said he sometimes could understand, much as shamans know the language of the birds. Less sophisticated cases gave him no trouble, nor did the wooden dumbness so often met with in divided selves under interrogation. In Haiti, as I have recounted in *The Invisibles*, this affliction is held to be the work of a Loa called Great Tree and is dealt with by the usual method of ritual incubation.[10] Laing needed much less time. As witness, a video was made during his appearance at a Milton Erickson conference. He offered to have a normal conversation, in public, with anyone diagnosed as schizophrenic, deemed intractable, and not under medication. Introduced to a homeless woman who fitted this bill, Laing so engaged her attention that after an hour she agreed to continue the conversation before a large audience, which she did with aplomb. Laing said that he had no technique in achieving this result. It was, he insisted, the result of empathy in the service of co-presence, the state of mind I have already alluded to by way of my quotations from Coleridge and Coventry Patmore.

But an ability to empathise can be perilous. I met him one morning, looking ghastly. Ghastly was a word frequently on his lips at the time and yes, he said, that's how it was with him. He'd woken up from a dream in which he'd been a rat in a Hong Kong sewer. He was in much the same state at one of the weekly Philadelphia Association meetings, which I will give a brief account of, if only in order to give you an idea of what I mean by a "shamanic temperament". Instead of getting on with the agenda, Laing asked if we would help him, for he was in a peculiar state. He felt like exploding and breaking the furniture. As it was, he was filled with this dire impulse down to his feet, which he wiggled for the next hour to free them from cramps.

Knowing something of that state, I offered to give his feet a massage by way of emergency treatment, which he indignantly refused. Just as well. He might have kicked my teeth in had I tried. Hugh Crawford then offered to put him through a formal inquisition, which Laing accepted by sliding off his chair onto the floor. First question: What brought it on? Laing replied that he'd just returned from Rome (this was the time when he'd refused to meet the Pope), and he and an Israeli doctor who, like himself, had a consuming interest in (here his voice faltered) foetuses, were sharing a bottle in a hotel bar. The doctor remarked, "Look at that woman, she's a Coca-Cola woman." Laing looked up, took her in at a glance and went off to vomit.

"Why," he asked of no one in particular, "do I take all this in? It lodges in my throat like a vampire." He was, he said, exsanguinated by it all. It must be because his umbilical cord had been cut as soon as he was born, much too early, his mother having already dissociated herself from his existence.

"That's a condensation," Crawford said. Laing ignored him, and with tears streaming down his cheeks, told of the conflict raging between his two hemispheres. "I feel both of them," he said. "They alternate, I've seen them in detail in myself." A heterodyne effect, Crawford remarked. Yes, but what was it about? Laing gave the answer: it had to do with an incorrigible evil in himself that waited on the incorrigible necessities of life in general.

"Regard the condensation," Crawford continued. Laing obliged, adding that he could go on like this for months. He knew it all. Crawford persisted until, grateful though I was to have heard what Laing confided to us while under this interrogation, I lost patience and attacked Crawford ad rem. Leaving the foetal issue to look after itself, I asked if he didn't recognise a mild case of shamanic disorder when he saw it: the moment when the gearbox is seized up and one can't shift either up or down, or know how to re-stimulate the works without further recourse to analytic procedure?

Crawford feigned not to understand. "You speak air," he told me. Laing broke in, "I breathe with my brain," he said, "I learnt to do that in order not to die during an asthma attack." Crawford, "That's a metaphor. You breathe with your lungs." This scientistic remark infuriated me. I got on his case once more, and so we slang each other for a time. Energised by this brawl, Laing soon joined in to slang Crawford on his own terms. He was now back in his chair with his gearbox unjammed, his hemispheres having found a common axis with his witness and spinning like a top. But what was his incorrigible evil, then asked Leon Redler. "Callousness," he replied, after a brief pause, and enlarged on that topic for a while. He was himself again.

Yes, Laing could be callous, and often was. It was, at best, part of his armamentarium against Coca-Cola women and the like; at worst, brutal. But then, we all have our little problems, do we not, complete with their own thick skins? Better to return to this account of a mild shamanic disorder by saying how much my contribution owed to that Brazilian I spoke of earlier, whose ability to shift gear caught my attention when I first met him. This was just before one of his shamanic performances, when he was so self-absorbed I thought him autistic. An opinion that what he later told me of his childhood did something to confirm, as did his successful treatment of autistic children. (Here then may be another diagnostic category by which to understand the shamanic crisis.) But he had discovered how to move in and out of this self-preoccupation: he went into first gear, if somewhat reluctantly, when I introduced myself to him, then into second when an attractive woman joined in, and into third when it was time for him to start his act. Then the spirit of the late emperor Nero (one of many that attended him) came into him and up he rose, like a spring, his face transformed, to work the audience and attend to his victim-patient. And he had a fourth gear ready for those moments when, having gone as far as he knew by himself, Messalina would animate his place of self-witness at his expense, to do the necessary in a flash. But the great difference between him and Laing was that I never saw Laing lose self-witness, let alone indulge in such histrionics, even though he did acknowledge that some of his best moments were inspired by a clearheaded Kali-esque furore. But that was later, when he had abandoned the Philadelphia Association.

I have so far spoken but indirectly of shamanic healing. This is a subject difficult to do justice to in a few words, since it deals with spells, curses, breaches of taboo, underhand intentions, social dysfunction, soul-loss and other anthropological commonplaces, many of which have escaped psychiatric attention. The methods used to free the victim of such complaints are much the same the world over: shamans must establish a reflexive world animated by personifications of the forces active in this one, and employ their empathic sense to discern which personifications of spirit are involved in a particular disorder. This done, various arts of conjuration are employed to so fascinate the attention that the patient is freed from self-preoccupation and can re-establish normal relations with the world at large. The methods are not always gentle, and some shamans are notable for their intimate knowledge of sadomasochistic necessities.

Practices of this kind, along with religions, can be distinguished according to whether they follow the affirmative or the negative way, and traditional shamanism largely favours the affirmative one. Laing's method, as practised in the households of the Philadelphia Association, favoured the negative way, as befitted his minimalist and existential bent. His guiding line was the Hippocratic oath with its major injunction to do no harm to those who consult you, to which he added his own gloss, that a human being should be treated as a human being and not suffer the consequences of being pathologised, whatever the problem. Hence his refusal to set up a conventional regimen by which sufferers can be restrained and manipulated, and his horror of the unconvivial nature of psychiatric wards. A horror so large that, as I have mentioned, he constantly extolled conviviality as the eminent need for those in mental shipwreck.

His view of the households set up by the Philadelphia Association was that they provided asylum, and "asylums" was often his name for them. They had no resident therapists, the task of running a household being taken up by the residents themselves, who sometimes included apprentices. There was no prescription of drugs, and if someone should freak out, the residents were expected to form a safety net on their own, and call on other households to help if necessary, with those who had oversight of these concerns also lending a hand.

There were no rules in the formal sense of the word. The asylum was also a crucible in which, Laing used to say, rough edges were smoothed out little by little. An odd kind of crucible, I once remarked, with no cross marked on its bottom, at which pedantry he pshawed in reproof. No cross and no apparent limits either. Instead, he appealed to the golden rule: to do nothing to others you would not like done to yourself, along with two others I once heard him appeal to, to make up for the lack of formal limits. One went:

What is not forbidden is allowed
What is not allowed is forbidden

whose rigour was mercifully put into question by the second rule: It's all up for grabs. These rules generally kept things in order and it was in this inchoate theatre, with no director, no script, no prompter, no stage props or effects, no drums or rattles, no invocations, prayers, chants and mind-altering brews, that the Laingian mode of spontaneous self-becoming could achieve the same general effects that are produced by shamanic initiation – of regression into nightmare, of its incubation, with a frenzy or two before the novice comes back into their senses with reintegrated faculties. The particular effects, however, were different, for no shamans were produced by this set-up. That was not the aim of the venture, which was to allow a mental disorder to be fully experienced as it ran its course, this being enough to ensure its happy outcome, no policing required. He was not interested in curing a disorder, I once heard him say, but in healing those distressed by disorder. In other words, he gave them their natural due, the chance to wise up to themselves by themselves.

I have but some further stories to tell you, to show Laing in action. The first concerns myself when I had a painful choice to make and could not see my way. I telephoned him one evening, asking for his help. All right, he said wearily, come over, and soon I was in that dark green room of his, telling him all about it. He bore with me patiently for quite a while, then got up and began walking to and fro in front of the curtains, back stooped, gesturing with his hands, eyes staring at nothing, silently jawing away non-stop. Alarmed by this parody of myself, my mind then cleared and I burst out laughing, whereupon he sat at his piano, opened a book of Noel Coward's songs, and so we passed the rest of a now convivial evening. I reminded him of the occasion years later, and he said – a little reproachfully, I thought – that there were times he wished someone had done as much for him.

Next, that unusual occasion in which I first saw him publicly engage in his speciality, which he later called psychic aikido. In contrast to usual shamanic and vaudouistic practice, in which the practitioner uses their left hand alternately with their right – the right for white magic, in aid of a client, the left for black, to deal with the client's enemies – psychic aikido takes the client as their own worst enemy and launches the telling blow, by which hand makes no odds, at the solar plexus of the situation. In this case, however, Laing was dealing, not with a client, but with an established member of his own profession. This was Carl Rogers, who had invited Laing to put on a double act in London.[11] Laing had accepted and in return had offered Rogers his hospitality for the duration. He had meanwhile summoned the members and associates of the Philadelphia Association on the evening of his guest's arrival, who had come, I was surprised to find, with his own band. As surprising was the silence that reigned over the room when I entered it, which continued until Rogers took it as his duty, Laing showing no such willingness, to introduce himself and his doings, after which his followers did likewise. There was another silence which, thinking that Laing needed a Mutt to his Jeff, I broke by following suit, to be followed in turn by the others of Laing's *équipe* [team]. Silence once more, long but not too long. And then Laing launched his opening gambit: "I see that we can work together, but I don't think we can ever be friends."

Gasps. Rogers paled beneath his tan, and sat speechless. Not so his band, who were loud in outrage. When the clamour uneasily subsided, Laing proposed that, the meeting being over, we should all adjourn to the Chinese restaurant around the corner. He was there first, and seeing him installed with two others at a corner table already supplied with bottles, I took a seat elsewhere. Rogers came in next, and took the chair next to me ("Serves you right for acting the gentleman," Laing sneered afterwards.) We engaged in small talk, and he was recovering his spirits when, as we were eating our noodles, two drunken Scotsmen lurched through the door. Laing shouted a welcome to them in broad Glaswegian, adding "If you want to see a pairson, he's sitting over there," stabbing a finger in Rogers' direction.

Another hubbub arose, and the restaurant soon emptied. On my more leisurely return to Laing's house, I saw Rogers and his folk in anxious discussion on the other side of the street. Leaving them to it, I found Laing and some others at the window, looking down upon the scene with the relish St Augustine described as one of the chief pleasures of the blessed, namely, to observe the torments of the damned, a passage Laing knew by heart. However, when he judged that enough was enough, he supposed he should go over and rescue Rogers from himself, which he did.

Next morning, the double act did very well. Laing was impeccable when introducing Rogers as the founder of non-directive client-centred therapy, and in asking many an interesting question. For instance, "How was it, do you think, that your psychology caught on so quickly in the United States?", to which Rogers replied, I thought without guile, "I suppose I came along at the right time as a kind of a person or something."

You may wonder what all this was about. If so, you should read the account of Martin Buber's public I–Thou encounter with

Rogers, in Buber's *The Knowledge of Man*. Buber talked of such things as "imagining the real", which Rogers failed to appreciate, and of a therapeutic dialogue being bounded by tragedy because of which "Humanity, human will, human understanding, are not everything. There is some reality confronting us. We cannot forget it for a moment." Rogers agreed that "there is an objective situation there, one that could be measured," which will give you some idea of the difference between the two men. Buber's final comment (with which Laing would have concurred) was that Rogers' concept of persons was little better than one of individuals, and that he was against individuals and for persons. On the other hand, he later said that he had never before attempted an I–Thou encounter in public, and found it to be not as impossible as he had supposed.[12]

If only it had been Laing talking with Buber, Laing, for whom such public encounters came to be meat and drink! He would have known just how it was with Buber when he smashed a Bible on the table, crying "What is the use of a book like this to us now?!", the time being the Nazi era, the event a rabbinical convention. And Buber would have appreciated Laing's remark that there were many people who, though worthy, he could not educate even if he wished to, because they did not entertain him.

I would be going beyond my assignment were I to speak of Laing's activities as a master of psychic aikido at the time he was preaching unconditional love and being so unconditional in his treatment of others that, though they were at first appalled, they were soon effusive in their gratitude. Long before, I had occasion to bring up this unconditionality of his with Peter Mezan[13], and found myself saying that Laing was impossible, to which he replied, "Obstinately impossible," and then regaled me with his anecdote, whose tragic condensation brings me to a close. That morning, he had paid Laing a visit and found him entertaining a tall, thin Spaniard who, dressed in black, complete with cape and a slouch hat, was armed with an invitation to visit Madrid. There, Laing would be given the keys to the city and meet the king. "You are as god to us," said he. "No one has read your books, but we all want to meet you. We think of you as Jesus Christ, because you attempted the impossible and failed."

I don't know how Laing dealt with this challenge to his honour. What would you say, were you Odran redivivus, and your works available, to an admirer who excused his failure to do the possible by making you that gift of gifts, a crown of thorns?

FANTASY AND REALITY

I believe in individual freedom and in existential philosophy, even if not quite in liberal philosophy. My therapy doesn't involve techniques or a method. And there is no goal either. The therapist shouldn't have a goal. Therapy belongs to the Aristotelian practical sciences, and it is a big mistake that psychotherapy, psychology and psychiatry have long been pushing to be recognised as theoretical and productive sciences, to belong to the safe, regulated sector even though, with this move, they would lose the very essence of their being.[1]

As soon as psychology split off from psychiatry, it lost its way in the maze of Cartesian, Newtonian and Galilean mechanistic formulas. Now psychology examines reality only through these reductionist patterns. But after Einstein, this is Paleolithic psychology. Isolated objects in space that obey universal laws: this isn't physics, it's a totalitarian state. We are all similar, even homogenous as far as the state is concerned. Galilei's example is even more dangerous than Descartes. While Giordano Bruno, the speculating philosopher, was arrested, tortured and killed, Galileo Galilei just had to stay at home.[2] He could enjoy the fine wines of his cellar as long as he stayed silent. Bruno told us to be open to the possibility that there is an unlimited number of worlds, not just one. Many! Dictatorship can't exist! But we sided with Galilei, not Bruno.

In *Novum Organum,* Francis Bacon explains that science is only interested in things that would remain true even if there were no life, no consciousness.[3] A brilliant thought. Let's eliminate ourselves, or in other words, let's eliminate our world. Once we have managed to marginalise our world and our experiences, in theory it shouldn't take more than one step to eradicate everything that is alive. It is an illusion that we are separate, isolated things in time and space, in a world that is not like what we believe it to be. The state passes laws that apply equally to everyone. We can be ruled by computers, only logic matters. No need to think. Bacon also speaks about nature as a lady whose secrets science wants to find and solve. At one time, nature was a goddess, the mother-goddess in whose womb we all lived. But now we live outside nature, we look at her from the outside, objectifying her with our stare. This lady, according to Bacon, is free: she is free to do whatever she likes. We want to catch her and restrict her, tie her down into a chair and torture her until she gives up all her secrets. Just as we used to torture witches to confess the truth. There is no love in this. Man against nature/woman.

We need a new paradigm. We need to make space for human consciousness. Our equations reflect reality and reality reflects our equations. How come? Reality is a dual unity (the mind and the world), not a schizoid duality (the world without the mind). Isolated individuals sewn into leather sacks, who all have to move according to one law, is a hallucination. A lot of patients start seeing a psychologist or psychiatrist because they have managed to break out of this false paradigm but have not yet found a companion outside this fallacy. They are not able to integrate their experiences yet. They can't go back to where they used to be, and they have not arrived to the other side yet. A shipwreck. We won't help them by pulling them back to where they used to be, to the inhumane, dead, Galilean world. If we have not managed to break free of this old scientific nightmare, how can we help those who have already broken free? Those who break out of this prison are faced with very real, genuine dangers. Psychiatrists are sometimes more scared of consciousness, of the mind, than anything else. Psychophobia is a fear of the mind, of consciousness or the human soul, whether our own or others'. Psychiatrists are terrified of becoming patients because they know what will happen to them.

Still, there is hope. This world always has sages, wise people, who have innocent, simple knowledge of what should be done. Simple is often very difficult: meditation, for example. To see reality as it is. Every tradition is a kind of ignorance, or in other words, a kind of sin, just not a Christian sin. The Bible says, "To be sure, sin was in the world before the law was given, but sin is not charged against anyone's account where there is no law."[4] To believe in Christian law is the greatest sin, or ignorance, Christians can commit. This is why many of them are judgemental and unkind. Love and compassion are the path, not alienated and alienating science.

Psychotherapy has the following elements: a therapist, a patient, a regular appointment and a reliable place. These things are not difficult to organise. The real challenge is for two people to actually meet at the set time and space. According to Laing, "Psychotherapy must remain an obstinate attempt of two people to recover the wholeness of being human through the relationship between them."[5]

Unheard-of simplicity; professional heresy. Only the patient matters. Protocol, regulations, the rules of theoretical science don't matter. Therapy is a primary here-and-now experience with the therapist and the patient both taking part. The experience is always fresh and alive. It is different with each patient. Treatment is exactly how we, people, treat each other; how we deal with each other. I go to the patient, to the human being. I don't ask them to come to where others are (the normal, the healthy, the successful, the rich, the beautiful, the parents, the teachers, the neighbours, the bosses, the husbands, the wives or the strangers). I don't leave them alone. I am there with them. I encourage them not to be afraid, or even if they are afraid, to be able to overcome their fear. The patient is searching for their own path and I don't know what their path is; that's something only they can know. Therapy is the process by which patients find their own path.

Why does this person, my patient, sit here across from me? Because they are suffering. They have admitted that they are suffering. Only those who admit they are suffering can become patients. And why do I sit here across from them? Why am I a therapist? Experience tells us that no one suffers without being hurt by someone. There is a deep covenant between the therapist and the patient, and they work together until the patient realises what kind of circumstances, people and environment they need to live, to become the person they really are. Suffering doesn't necessarily decrease in the course of therapy but the patient learns to tolerate it. They learn to easily and cheerfully coexist with suffering. The terrible thing has already happened to all of us, so the therapist and the patient are suffering together. The best therapists started their careers as patients. Laing was once asked, during a Q&A session, how he managed to get to the point where he was not suffering any more. Laing's eyes opened wide in disbelief. He couldn't comprehend how someone could ask such a stupid question. "A therapist is not one who doesn't suffer but one who suffers well," he said.

Every child wants to cure their parents so they can be loved in a way that is good for them. But there are some children who don't succeed. Maybe they are the ones who become therapists. According to Lipót Szondi, only those people become real therapists who had at least one lunatic in their family.[6] If you live with a lunatic, you die, go crazy or learn how to survive the situation. It's sink or swim. The patient is not an object to be fixed but a person to accept. If they were an object, they could be described, they would have characteristic measurements, there could be a test that would detect any discrepancy between them and the average, the normal. A broken arm can be set in a cast according to a template, but therapy can't have a template. I don't examine my patients; I live with them. The patient needs desireless loving attention to understand what their own real desires are. They got lost because they played roles, because they wanted to live according to others' expectations, because they had to fulfil others' desires. Tigers and fish need different things. It takes time for the person who comes to therapy to become revealed. You can't hasten the development of a relationship. I can't rush to love you to fulfil a deadline. According to Sándor Ferenczi, a good therapist is someone with lots of time and no ambition.[7] There is no "you" and "I," no isolation or separation, there is only "us," all of us, all in the same boat.

At first, we might have to admit that the only real experience as we are sitting together is the absence of our relationship.

Nowadays, the most frequent thing people suffer from is alienation from themselves, from each other and from the world, so much so that we almost accept it and consider it normal. Those who are not able or willing to accept their designated life are regarded as ill or abnormal. We have treatments for them and stuff them full of medication so their crying or raving is not too noisy. Therapy looks for the roots of alienation; it sheds light on the little games our parents, school or society, forced us into before we had the power to defend and protect ourselves. Therapy is successful when the patient breaks free of the straitjacket of roles that have been forced on them.

Once I worked with a married couple, and we were talking about their son, a 23-year-old man. He still lived with them and the parents were afraid of some violent, fierce explosion because he had already threatened both his father and mother. They thought of locking him up or sending him to prison because they were scared of him. "I don't want to see him hurt, except through a doctor!" sobbed his mother, with an Eastern European accent. I have heard several parents express their views that it would be better for their child to be sick or mad than to risk finding out some secret or terrible truth.

When we lose the relationship with the spirit that keeps us alive, the spirit that we are all unified in and that we are only tiny particles of, we also lose the experience of ecstasy. All that is left are the daily chores, the tasks and the tedious misery of survival.

Therapy must continue until we find the experience that is the origin of all religions: we are not isolated separate entities crippled in our wretched skin-encapsulated egos. We belong together and there is a common consciousness or spirit that needs us. We are all drops of water in a great wave, we flow in and through each other and we blend with each other. We are never alone.

I would be bored if I couldn't get close to my patients. Jerzy Kosinski once said there is only one game worth playing in life: how close can I get to someone without anybody getting hurt or injured.[8] As soon as I heard this, I knew right away that it was my game. It is extremely difficult for me to understand why so many people protect themselves against this. Laing said it was psychophobia: the terror of our own and other people's minds, souls.

According to Freud, one's character will have formed by the age of three.[9] I think this is only true if we take "character" not as the unchangeable self, but as an accumulation of habits we develop over a number of years to be able to survive our families. The good news is that there is no habit we can't get rid of. We don't actually have a character; we only have habits. There is no personality development because there is no personality. It doesn't take much to hunt down animals with habits that are easy to know, but a real fighter, a warrior, never has any habits. They are unpredictable.

There are automatic, recurring experiences, emotions, thoughts and associations. In meditation, these can become spontaneous experiences, springing from the heart, from the present. Science is always about recurring things that can be described and validated. One's habits are not like this because they can be changed. Gravity is not a habit. This doesn't mean that, if I am aware of my habits, I will want to get rid of them, and even if I did, it is not necessarily going to be easy. When I attended therapy with Laing, I compiled a long list of all my habits, ticked those that served me well and got rid of those that didn't. When we get to know the works of an artist, for example, we know that this is a Cézanne, this is a Van Gogh, etc., their so-called style is really just pieced together from the habits of the artist. The world expects an accomplished artist to have recognisable habits, but this has nothing to do with art. I can imagine an artist who is not recognisable by their work because each painting starts from scratch, without habits or a familiar style.

In my first psychology course, I was told that the goal of psychology is to predict and control human behaviour.[10] I thought I had wound up in a lunatic asylum where everyone was in a delusional daze. But, I had to pretend to be asleep with them, otherwise I wouldn't have gotten my diploma.

We shouldn't underestimate the power of habits. We are sleeping, sleepwalking, and in our sleep our habits automatically move instead of us. We can very quickly transform our environment to suit our habits. In our new family, or at our new workplace, we soon start to have the same experiences as at our childhood home. To achieve this, we naturally need partners, co-sleepers who allow us to pull them into the roles we assign them. But fortunately, there are some who don't allow themselves to be pulled in. There are bosses who say, "Hey, I am not your father, stop acting like this." We should surround ourselves with such people. The environment and the community are always responsible for what I am doing if they allow me to do it and if they don't tell me that something is not right. I am fortunate if I wake up from my sleepwalking because there are consequences. If you feel hurt, you might ask, "How could you do this to me?" But you'd have to add, "And how could I let you?" We can stop each other from going crazy by saying, "Hey, don't do that." If the other person prefers to stay asleep and instead of waking up, runs away, then, well, what can you do? You can't wake someone up if they don't want to wake up; the only thing you can do is not sing a lullaby when they momentarily wake up. When a teenager wakes up for a moment, the whole family starts singing that they really don't want to talk about whatever is happening. If someone wakes up in a group of sleeping people, everyone will be mad at them. This is what happened with Christ, so they put him to sleep forever.

In light of all this, we can easily see that there are certain concepts and words that don't mean anything, for example, "self-knowledge". Well, that term is total bullshit. We could even think that "I", as a person, can get to know "me", a person. It's as if there are two people and one is examining, walking around, undressing, dissecting, scanning, analysing and trying out the other person. A veritable Punch-and-Judy show. Then, when they have got to know them, they can relax and start living because the future no longer holds any secrets. There is a huge issue here though, which is the obvious incongruity of pretending that I am two people. Where does this lie, this hallucination, come from? Where did I get the idea that I can separate me from myself? How can I lie to myself when that is also an impossibility? How can I hide what I know from myself? "Language is a virus from outer space," says William S. Burroughs.[11] Language hypnotises us all. We think something exists because there is a word for it. We say "unicorn", but that doesn't mean that unicorns definitely exist. Self-knowledge is discussed a lot, it is developed in training courses, but it is an absurdity, a logical paradox. Actually, this word immediately takes us over the threshold of madness.

According to my definition, madness is when we lose touch with reality, and here, language distances us from reality rather than taking us closer. What does this word "self-knowledge" do? It doubles us. It creates a duality of consciousness. I get to know myself. Let's just consider this! One of my selves starts chatting with the other, getting to know him. We start our lives as objects because our mothers, fathers and others treated us as objects. They talked about us as objects in our presence, in third person singular (he, she, they). We take this perspective on without noticing how absurd it is because we don't yet have the mental ability to resist. We become an object before becoming a subject, even though we can only have actual experiences from the perspective of the subject (not in language). That is the only real perspective. When I claim to be thinking about myself and my own experiences, when I examine, analyse and get to know myself, the object, then I am actually pretending to be someone else: my mother, my father or another person who is looking at me. When we look at ourselves as objects, what we are actually doing is pretending that we are not alone. It is nothing but a false duality. We are sucking our thumbs so we don't get scared by being entirely on our own.

It is true that there are desires, thoughts, feelings, phenomena and experiences, and it is also true that constantly, at every second, I am at crossroads where I can make a choice. Will I take my experiences seriously? What will I pay attention to? What commitments will I make? What priorities should I have? How will I design the hierarchy of things? How are things constituted? What am I going to do? I will never be able to discover whether I am brave or not at a "self-knowledge" course. But I can go off to battle or embark on a challenging and risky venture, and I will be sure to find out. If I decide that I will be "the brave person", or in other words, I want to prove that I am brave in novel situations, then I have to practise being brave. That's the only solution. Tests, self-analysis, or a full blood count will not reveal whether or not I am brave.

If I appear brave in various situations, then sooner or later others will say, "Now, that's a brave person". This is a label that has nothing to do with my future, it's just a reward for my past. There are certain labels we are happy to wear: brave, intelligent, strong, diligent, honest; and there are other labels that we don't like to wear: lazy, cowardly, stupid, inept. But the mere existence of these labels doesn't predestine my future actions to conform to any of them. And if my free will can influence what I am going to do in the next moment, then I can obviously pick up or drop these labels as I wish. This is what I think is worth knowing about so-called "self-knowledge".

What good does it do that this fashionable and meaningless expression is so popular? Why is it good, and who benefits from believing that there is such a thing as self-knowledge, even though a few minutes of precise thinking is sufficient to understand that it is an absurdity? Linguistic traps and labels all originate from the community or society. They express the needs of the community. If the community needs lots of daring hunters in the tribe, then it is sufficient to tell a boy that he is a brave hunter after his first lucky hunt, and from that time onwards, the tribe will respect him and he will get all the facilities associated with his status. The problems start when, for some reason or another, the needs of the community dictate that we don't discover there is trouble in the community, in the family or in our society. Piecemeal solipsism transfers to the individual from the communal, the problems between people and the area of trying to resolve them. "Work on yourself, develop yourself, and once you achieve the 'required stage', your life will change as well." "Don't try to work out whether you like it in this family, or what's wrong in this school or community." "Don't pay attention to who your friends are (everyone who has your interests at heart in a way that is good for you), who your enemies are (everyone who is not your friend), but learn self-knowledge, map out your shortcomings and sort them out." "Work on yourself!" prevents revolutions, discourages solidarity, and creates the false ideal that I should be able to rise above my circumstances, no matter how oppressive, injurious or crazy-making they are.

Fleeting fashion will, however, die out on its own. Since the age of about 30, I've been inspired by the eternal, by that which already existed for Plato, Socrates, Montaigne and Pascal. Friedrich Wilhelm Nietzsche hated those who oscillated between satisfaction and resentment. They are people who chicken out of real life because it fluctuates and flows forcefully between curses and blessings, crying and laughing. Laing inspired me with the belief that authentic life exists and one doesn't have to pay with conformity to be part of it. I was inspired by the revolution of emancipation, solidarity and compassion. These are more relevant today than ever before. These are eternal signposts.

I have an ethical responsibility not to allow others to project their father or mother onto me. One shouldn't succumb, shouldn't allow others to treat them as if they were someone else. One major difference between Laing and most other psychoanalysts is how he dealt with transference. My first analyst, a traditional Freudian-trained analyst, made me lie back on a couch, he sat behind me so I couldn't see him and he hardly ever spoke. He transformed himself into a blank screen and I could project onto him my mother, my father or anyone I wanted. With Laing, I sat across from him, we had deep discussions and he was totally himself, so it was impossible to project my mother, my father or anyone else onto him. As soon as I tried, he made fun of me. In this way, one can get rid of transference much more quickly. I am responsible for being spontaneous and honest, for telling the other person to their face when they are venturing away from reality. Madness is nothing but losing our connection with reality. Once I went to see one of my professor colleagues at a university and told him that, if he makes everyone working for him scared, people will be afraid of him, no one will tell him the truth and he will become increasingly idiosyncratic, like a runaway engine without a governor. I took responsibility for telling him the truth, for telling him what he was doing. The Greek term *parrhesia* means to speak truth to power. A parrhesiast might start with, "Don't kill me, but the truth is that…". One can always practise courage.

At one point in my life, I spent a lot of time reading mad people's autobiographies. Looking back, they could clearly see, and could even describe in accurate detail, that they were at their craziest when they were the most certain of themselves, someone or something. One of the most interesting is the memoir of Daniel Paul Schreber.[12] By writing his autobiography, Schreber became the most well-known paranoid schizophrenic of the 19th century. Freud made a detailed analysis of his case. Schreber described his first suspicions that his experiences might not mean what he was so sure they did. In his consciousness, divine rays were tormenting his body and they were penetrating his ass. Today, we know how normal his suspicions were. As it turned out, Schreber's father, Moritz Schreber, was a doctor who worked out a precise system of "black pedagogy" and tested it on his sons. He concocted equipment for improving posture that worked by viciously stabbing the child's body if the required ideal posture was relaxed, even for a moment. Papa Schreber's system was built on corporal punishment, pain and humiliation. After the thrashing, the child had to shake his father's hand and thank him for the chastisement. Moritz Schreber's other son committed suicide in his thirties. Daniel Paul spent his life in various institutions, sometimes locked up, sometimes not, and he struggled with divine rays and sounds. After a while, however, he started having reservations about his own experiences. Later, in his memoir, he described how he started coming out of madness when he began to doubt what he was totally convinced of before.

Anxiety dulls one; it narrows one's consciousness. Men experience deeper separation anxiety than women; they often feel more cut off than women. Men will often become assholes because they are anxious. Being alone is so painful and terrifying that they don't have any capacity left to notice what else is there. When a man experiences this tension, he will look for tranquilisers, which he will find mainly in sex. A lot of men regard women as potential sex partners because they are terrified of not being able to do anything in their desperate loneliness. For an anxious man with a constricted consciousness, each woman is a wall socket, a hole, and he feels that if he can't stick his cock into that hole, his batteries will go dead. He would stick his cock into anything or anyone. This is totally impersonal. In fact, men don't even need a woman for this. They need electricity, that's why they jerk off, and that's what porn is for. These are all sedatives but they only treat the symptoms. It's like taking an aspirin for a headache; it doesn't treat the cause of the headache. Separation anxiety can only be treated by a real connection with a real person, or even with the universe. In the history of human evolution, women have spent a lot more time with children than men. Women's work was inside, while men worked outside. Interactions with children happen on an emotional level, not on a logical one. To deal with the world, one needs logic and detachment, while inside one needs personal dealings with children instead of logic. Children demand personal connection.

I often quote the last line of E.E. Cummings' poem, titled "i am so glad and very", where he says "i am through you so i."[13] This refers to not having a fixed, definitive I. Buddhists also believe that there is no self, no ego, and everything depends on the circumstances. The individual doesn't possess sexuality. It's not true that some people have a high libido and others a low one. Sex always manifests *between* people. That's why it is so important whom I choose as my partner; my sexuality depends on who I am with. The important thing is not the other person's performance or my performance, but how attractive and exciting they are to me and I am to them. If, during sex, my focus is on my performance, that's already far off the mark. But if the other person is more important than me, then we will both get something amazing out of it. So we must find a stupefyingly exciting lover who is more exhilarating than the pressure to perform. Again, rather than knowing oneself, it is getting to know the other person that is stimulating. This is getting to know what we can become together; the new us. At the age of 80, Carl Whitaker, the founder of family therapy, once whispered in my ear, conspiratorially, that he was rushing home to his wife. But it was not the woman herself that he was missing, rather the "us" he experienced with her. If his wife died, he would miss the "us" more than her.

Why is this "us" not obvious? In his book, *The Duality of Human Existence*, David Bakan speaks about our most basic duality: community existence (*communion*) and individual action (*agency*).[14] Every living thing, even a one-cell organism, exists in this duality. Everything the living entity does for themselves is *agency*, and everything they do to connect or communicate with others is *communion*.

It is good to have balance. "Self-knowledge", "self-development", "personality development" and other similar concepts tip the balance too much towards agency. We attribute too much competence to it. Bakan also writes about psychosomatic conditions. He considers cancer to be an illness of too much agency. Too much communion of course also creates problems when the individual places themself too much behind the community. In crisis situations, there is a great need for communion because everyone has to obey the commander; then it is alright to have hierarchy. That's why politicians love, and at times create crises; they are great at creating them because it is easier to govern within a hierarchy. In a crisis situation, we submit ourselves to the will of our superior. That doesn't happen during peaceful times. Simone Weil, out of great compassion, only ate her allotted rations in a starving France in 1942. She became weak and died. She was 34. This is an instance of too much communion and too little agency. I have already quoted Rabbi Hillel several times on the ethics of communion and agency, when he says "If I am not for myself, who will be for me? And being only for myself, what am I? And if not now, when?" So, agency is very important because only I know my experiences. We could even say only I know who I am. Each ant looks after itself. Each individual has to look after itself, but whatever extra energy I have, I can give to the community. That is how I maintain myself and maintain the community.

The big question, maybe the biggest, is: how do we deal with each other? How do I deal with the other person? What do I tolerate, and what do I not tolerate? How do I deal with myself, and what do I fight for? How to love and what to do with a bully?

According to Levinas, it is not enough to be responsible for myself; I am also responsible for the other's responsibility.[15] If I see someone hurting somebody and I do nothing, don't interfere, then I am wicked too. I am not moving to Syria to become a nurse but I can ask my neighbour not to scream at their kids. I also have to speak out if the neighbour, an official, or anyone, mistreats me.

If I just dedicate myself to others but don't look after myself, if I treat others well but don't pay attention to myself, expecting the communion, the community, to support me like a strong fabric, that will only work if everyone does the same. It is difficult to find balance. A mother will sacrifice everything; she will die for her child. Her baby is more important than herself. But for the sake of maintaining a balance, someone will have to take care of her, look after her. The father, the family and the community look after the new mother: she gets maternity pay, etc. The baby bites the mother's breast and she cries out. She doesn't let the baby do that. She doesn't actually give herself fully. She doesn't want to be hurt by her child. The other day, a young mother came to see me and told me that her five-year-old son punched her in the stomach so hard, she felt sick. She just told her son that she couldn't believe it. I asked her why she reacted in that way. If someone punched me in a dark alleyway, I'd punch them back, fall on the ground, call the police or run away if I could. I'd protect myself somehow. Whoever has agency will protect themself. The child who punches his mother has agency, but the mother who lets it happen doesn't. If I don't protect myself, if I don't make it clear that I have agency, then I turn the other person into a monster. That is also a responsibility.

We can be hurt and feel burning pain in our relationships with people, but if we try too hard to avoid pain, we'll end up a lonely recluse. After being hurt, you need courage to still be able to look for people who won't hurt you. Not everyone gets a chance to feel communion, to experience from the outset the feeling that it's wonderful to be a tiny part of something great. Before and after our birth, we are a tiny part of the great whole of our mother, this itself is communion. Some refer to it as *participation mystique*. The child's consciousness is not separated from the mother's consciousness for about nine months after birth and even later on, for years, the mother is the most important person in the child's life. If the child had a nice time in their mother and with their mother then, when they grew up, they will constantly look for communion because, within their experience, this miracle does exist. By merging into a communion, they can experience the joy of unity. On the other hand, if being in the mother was awful, and if unity with the mother was painful and terrifying, then they become afraid that it will be awful being with others too, and if it turns out to be nice, then they don't want to believe it. Or they might even want to ruin or destroy the other person or community who accepted them with love. The experience of a subsequent loving communion doesn't override the prior hell they had experienced with their mother or in their mother. The therapist's task is to provide an experience that proves people exist who are a pleasure to be close to. Being a therapist is a dangerous occupation.

We can't just have a cognitive experience that unity, love and communion are the reality. Communion or *co-presence* (being present with an other) is brought about by two or more people being together without any of them having to edit themselves or having to behave in a particular way to suit the others' expectations, to fit their script. In *co-presence,* each participant can give themself up to what is, to that thing which is greater and more than the sum of its constituent parts. There are no power games, no tyranny, no subservience and no surrender to the other person, no fusion. There is only uninhibited play, joy and unconditional belonging. John Heaton said that Ronnie could do this. When Ronnie entered a room, we glimpsed the sparkle of the possibility of human kindness. It was an experience, not an instruction. Where did this come from?

Laing took the Hippocratic oath very seriously in his heart, in his brain and everywhere; he didn't want to cause any harm. Somehow, this determination radiated from his eyes and his gestures. You can't learn or teach this. Using a mountaineering metaphor, he explained responsibility to me: the first climber is responsible for the second climber. If I have slipped and am just hanging off the other climber, if endangered, they have the right and duty to cut me free. Ronnie thought he would cut me off sooner than I would cut him off. I would rather risk both of us dying. According to Laing, that was only possible because I had not thought things through properly to understand what is right and what is wrong. So, it wouldn't be the goodness of my heart motivating my actions but the lack of consistent logic. Are there situations where communion is more important than an individual's life?

In therapy, I come across so many words that are just tools or part of power games and trickery or illusion. Because only the powerful can utter these words, the servant, the subordinate, the child cannot. One can read G.W.F. Hegel, Slavoj Žižek and Michel Foucault to learn about this.[16] Manipulation and word jugglery blur reality instead of clarifying it. We have a game, let's say football, and we make up some rules. Those who are playing agree on these rules. But we often forget that the game is just a game because one can enter a game and one can leave a game. If we agree that this is what we are going to play, then I happily consent. We can even play a sadomasochist game just like many couples do. But we have to be careful because if we forget that this is a made-up game, then we are in trouble. It is crucial to know when it's a game and when it's not. Society is football, our company and the military, but it's crucial to know what game we are playing. Animals have a clear distinction between playing, aggression and sex. Drawing blood or impregnating a female is not a game, and neither are lacerated skin and torn fur. When a dog exposes their belly lying on their back, they are saying, "Don't hurt me, we are just playing!" At one time, blushing might have indicated to us, "Stop! Draw back, don't ask me what you are asking! I don't know what you want but I can't play with what you're doing now!" Our society today expects obedience from us in so many ways: fight, work, pay your taxes, follow the rules, etc. It might be a bold thing to question when obeying is a game and when it is not. In war, on a ship and in survival situations, demanding obedience is critical. There is no time for discussion. There are only orders and efficiency. Today, the tendency is to play a constant game of survival situations; simply living is practically impossible. If we believe that this is the world and we are afraid of not playing, then we feel ashamed. Švejk knew that everything was a game and he played by working out how to break all the rules and still not get court-marshalled.[17] All this is connected to power, and we often forget, or it doesn't even occur to us, that all this is just a power game. If one is terrified of their boss and their boss's criticism, I suggest they imagine that they are their boss's boss and they are criticising him. This, however, becomes an impossible mission if I forget that I am just part of a game. Laing, in his book *The Politics of Experience*, explains that there is a power game in every family and a child who realises that their family is playing a game that hurts them becomes a naughty, troubling child. According to Laing, in some families, there is a horrible game going on but no one can talk about it and they aren't even supposed to know it's a game. People living in these families are often labelled schizophrenic. In therapy, you can talk about this as well. You can demystify this hellish game and can simply and calmly state who has done what to whom.

The great fantasy in therapy is that one who "knows" something can help others who don't. In reality, however, one can't really do much to make things better for someone else. There are only three things we can do to help: one is to give shelter; two is to give encouragement; and three is to demystify. Here, I follow the lead of David Smail.[18]

1. The therapist gives shelter, even for an hour, where there are no games like in the outside world (yes, there are some people who have never had that shelter, not even for one moment). The shelter is a safe space where no one will bother you, no one will nitpick or ask questions, and they leave you in peace but not alone.

It's a safe space where you don't have to feel ashamed for wanting to get rid of all responsibilities, at least for the time being. It's a space where you can rest awhile and without anyone rushing you. You can find the path out of the forest you are lost in.

2. The therapist gives encouragement. Just not being alone is encouraging. I can't lead you because that's for you to do based on what you will or will not do, what you do or do not want. You need courage even to voice, to say out aloud, what your actual real desire is. I can only encourage you to do this if I take you seriously, if I don't make fun of you, and if I don't criticise you. And the only way I can genuinely encourage you to work for fulfilling your desires is by practising it myself in your presence.

3. The therapist demystifies. You say: "This happened... "I am like this..., or "The problem with me is..." And the therapist will help you wake up from this self-deception. Then, without feeling guilty, you can tell the truth about "who did what, and who did what to whom". Sartre calls this "praxis" and he calls the blinding self-deception "process".[19] "I ended up in Canada": this is "process". "After my sixteenth birthday, my father gave me a chance to escape from my mother, from high school and from Hungary. I decided to take this opportunity despite my mother's objections": this is "praxis".

"Deserves": This is another fantasy, like the castle spinning around on a duck's leg or the dragon with seven heads.[20] This word exists but there is no real meaning behind it. In reality, I want something, and I get it, or I want something, and I don't get it. When someone has a lot of things and I don't, I can screw with reality and say that they deserved it and I didn't. As if a child deserves the birch twigs, the candy, the coal or the chocolate from Santa Claus.[21]

Are thoughts sinful? When someone comes to see me, I can almost immediately work out whether the person is a Catholic or a Jehovah's Witness because they deeply believe and accept that the sin of thought is the same as the sin of deed or action. This fantasy creates a huge burden for a person. What I think doesn't actually harm anyone but everything I do has an effect. That's why it is important to have the opportunity to carefully think about everything that comes to my mind and use clear thinking to consistently explore all components and the ethics of a particular mental phenomenon. It is just as important to be able to talk about our thoughts, even about our most scandalous and rebellious thoughts, as it is about our experiences. One of Jung's patients told him that she wanted to marry him. Jung didn't discourage her but engaged in discussing all the details of the proposal. Finally, the woman told him that she was sorry but she had actually changed her mind. They shouldn't send out wedding invitations after all.[22] If you are forbidden from talking about or contemplating your desires, you cannot learn about them and cannot control them. If I don't know something, that something can control me without me knowing. That's why it is important to welcome all my desires. Which desires I will act on, and when, is another question completely. I also want to know my children's desires. I want them to be able to talk about all their dreams and desires without feeling ashamed. Which of these desires I will or won't help to fulfil is, again, another question. Parents who don't even want to know what their kids want, don't know their children. It is not pleasant to say "no", but it is much better than not even having a clue about our children's desires.

After Buddha attained enlightenment under the bodhi tree, he had visions. He saw all those things Ronnie spoke about: he saw people killing, raping, hurting, and destroying each other. He saw everything but he just sat there and did nothing. He had to come to a point where he wasn't shocked by what his brain could come up with any more. Following the example of Buddha, we could let our thoughts come and go, and we could learn not to identify ourselves with any of the thoughts. Not with the sinful thoughts and not with the innocent ones. This detachment is Buddhism's great gift. So, Buddhism is therapeutic. It is healing. It says the same thing as Ákos Fodor's poem about the "3 negative words" – *nincs/semmi/baj* – or, in English, "there isn't/nothing/wrong". The meaning is "all's well", "there's no problem", and/or "there's nothing wrong", which is also how Buddhism reframes things.[23]

Thought, fantasy and imagination are all innocent and harmless. Of course, from another perspective, that is not quite true. There is a difference between fantasy and imagination. Winnicott clearly differentiated between the two, and so do I. Fantasy or daydreaming (the spoiler of life) is so enjoyable and absorbing that one escapes reality over and over by going to fantasy-land: in other words, one ends not doing anything. Imagination, on the other hand, lights the fire under one's ass. It inspires one to act, and this can be called a creative fantasy. A lot of people believe the fantasy that, with the power of their imagination, they can attract things from the universe. But in reality, it is our actions, powered by the force of our imaginations, that can actually change reality. If I want to give a piano concert at Carnegie Hall, it is not enough to lie in bed and imagine it over and over again. I have to start learning and practising the piano very diligently. This "law of attraction" is nothing but superstition and megalomania: I think that my will is so powerful that I can control the powers of the universe. Oneness with the universe is not an illusion. It is possible to experience it and a lot of people have described it. I have also experienced it several times. Once, I was walking on the beach in an altered state of consciousness and I saw a dog. I could feel oneness and I thought, OK, now I will attract this dog. I expanded myself and called the dog in my thoughts. And the dog was happily wagging its tail, racing around the beach and showed no intention of obeying my will. The point here is that the dog and I are actually one but there is no individual will in oneness. That is why, as I have mentioned earlier in this book, Marion Milner often says the only real and proper function of one's will is wanting to not want.[24] I and the dog are parts of the *greater,* and that's the will that counts; that's the will I have to give myself over to. I think the dog already knows this even without having thoughts. That's what I think about the "law of attraction".

It is very painful to become aware of the minuteness of our existence. We are rowing in a tiny little boat in the middle of a great ocean and we can't even see the shore. But we would like to believe that we have control, we row here and there, we look into binoculars and we try to be clever. But all this only works as long as the water is calm, and although we have our suspicions, we would rather not think about this fact. We like to think just like a child does, that if we behave well, we will have a good life and nobody will hurt us. We pretend to have that power. This is our defence mechanism in the face of our insignificance. Can everyone become a Mozart? Hell, no! This is why Susan Sontag's book, *Illness as Metaphor*, is so important.[25] She fights everyone who thinks that she created or attracted her own breast cancer. They can all go and fuck themselves as far as she is concerned. Breast cancer is enough trouble for her. She wasn't going to allow the blaming of the victim.

We have to be very careful with what is true and what is not true. Lacan clearly explains that reality exists but it is so infinitely great and so complex that we will never be able to know it exhaustively.[26] Like in theology, God is more than what any word or sentence can express; no words can describe him. And in this terrifying infiniteness and minuteness, there is imagination, language and logos. We humans exist in the context of these three. We constantly fantasise about reality; our experiences are always a particular mixture of reality and imagination. The only thing that connects us is language. If we use it well, it strips away imagination from reality, but if we misuse language, it covers reality over with imagination. It will veil reality from us. The most important task of a psychotherapist is to strip away the veils. According to Wittgenstein, language can drive us mad and his philosophy is the therapy. If it is possible to talk about something, we should talk about it accurately, and if something can't be talked about, it's best to shut up. He demonstrates this in his book *Tractatus*.[27] He speaks clearly about the things that can be talked about and shuts up about the things that cannot be talked about. When I say you can't hurt or help someone with thoughts or imagination, I don't mean we can't empathise or resonate with each other. We flow through each other and into each other, but we don't control each other. Will is different from empathy. There is no will in empathy. That's why it's important for the therapist not to want anything but to give the experience to the patient that it is possible to be with someone without the other person wanting anything. People often run away from relationships because they don't know any relationship where the other person doesn't want anything.

Let's extend the tiny little boat metaphor. Let's imagine I wake up and find myself in this boat. I know the dangers, as I am in a fairly extreme situation, after all. It's all very desolate. What should I do now, knowing how infinitely tiny and insignificant everything is? Anyway, that's the life I have, so how should I live? Human thought has provided various answers to this question. The stoics of antiquity, Seneca and Epictetus, believed that death was better than a lot of things; it is not compulsory to live. In those days, there were men who kept poison in their belly buttons, and they lived by this motto: "If the room gets too smoky, you always have the back door. No need to be stuck inside!" These people were not afraid of anything because they were ready to die at any moment, so they couldn't be punished or held responsible.[28] Heidegger's categories of *vorhanden* and *zuhanden* are terminology for using what we have at hand, for paying attention to that without contemplating or theorising.[29] I have a look, see what I can touch, who my neighbour is, who is rowing the other boat, I play with the water, I stick my hand in the water and play with it until I die. Other people are rowing around me so, every so often, I hop over into other boats and we make love. Well, that's something worth living for. I am rowing north, so the shore will come sooner or later, the Messiah will come. This can also give meaning to life. It is us who give meaning to our lives. Someone deciding something is just as good as any other deciding anything else. If someone wants to become a doctor, that's good, or if they want to become a watchmaker, that's also good. Victor Frankl wrote from Auschwitz that those who couldn't give meaning to their lives died, but those who could find something to live for, even there, if they could help others, or anything, found it easier to survive.[30]

Nothing has any meaning in itself; we create all meaning. Ad absurdum, even if someone wants to live outside the law, that's also fine. In reality, there will be some people who identify with them and others who give meaning to their lives by pursuing them. At least they can play the cops-and-robbers or prison game.

The question comes up of what we should take seriously and what we should not take seriously. The Greeks were very good at demonstrating this duality in tragedies and comedies; either you cry or you laugh. Life is either a tragedy or a comedy. As far as I'm concerned, I would rather laugh. This whole thing is so absurd that one is forced to laugh. Laing had a capacity to laugh at anything and everything. Once, one of his friends had a great emotional problem in a relationship with a woman, and he went to see Laing for consultation. He was walking up and down, explaining his problem. He was up to his neck in the dilemma. Then he suddenly looked at Laing, who was walking up and down in the exact same posture, imitating him, waving his arms, gesturing and gesticulating. For about a minute, the friend looked at him in shock. What the hell was he doing? Then he burst out laughing and they spent the rest of the hour laughing.

For some reason, we take difficulties more seriously than easy things. Birds find it easy to overcome difficulties or burdens. If one is flying in one's dream, that means they are getting rid of their mother's bonds; mother earth's gravity is not pulling them down any more. This is also the best metaphor for good sex: one person is one wing, the other person is the other wing, and if they stick themselves into each other, together they can fly. This is good sex. One can't do it (fly) alone.

How can I deal with myself without forgetting that I am a sanctified being, a sacrament? How can I take myself seriously and how do I know who I really am, beyond all the influences of family and culture? What attracts my attention when no one is telling me what to pay attention to? Maybe that's what defines my individuality. Whatever guides me is my sacredness and maybe my attention takes me to the world that's mine. Francis Huxley said that you should notice what you pay attention to when you are free and then you should pay attention to what you noticed. There may be a genetic or spiritual predetermination to my fate because we don't all pay attention to the same thing. Each person has their individual interests and curiosity. There are children who pay attention to machines and devices; others are interested in spiders, colours, materials, and some others in sounds and tunes. If each child could get what they are really interested in, if their families and schools took them seriously, and if there wasn't an effort to fit them into schematic formulas, they could grow up absorbed in the *flow*. This is important, because happiness is a side effect of *flow*, as defined by Mihaly Csikszentmihalyi.[31]

So, I cannot become part of someone else's life or consciousness just by willing to be part of it. It doesn't work that way. But still, there is something. After an experiment, Duncan Blewett described an interesting phenomenon.[32] Twelve people locked themselves in a room. They all took LSD and they sat in a circle facing the wall, with their backs to each other. They all felt sick, they were moaning, and they didn't even want to look at each other. One of them finally spoke up and asked if someone would go out and throw up. And so, somebody did go out and vomited, and then they all felt better. So, willpower had a role to play here: they wanted someone to go out. Somebody had to say it, but everybody felt it. They were all different but they could all feel each other. There was no ego there anymore; everything was simultaneous. So, it is true that we are separate, but we are all one at the same time. And the calmer I am, the more calming influence I will have on my environment. The more agitated I feel, the more I'll agitate the other person. Laing was an excellent therapist because he didn't get agitated. He wasn't afraid. Young men quite often end up in psychiatric care because people get scared of them, but after half an hour the scary youth is not scary anymore. A good old therapist, like a midwife, doesn't get scared. They are not afraid. This feeling flows into the therapist's patient, or in the case of a midwife, into the mother giving birth, and everything becomes easier. But those who cover up their feelings drive everyone around them mad. I had a patient who felt extreme fear. She panicked whenever she was sitting in a car next to her husband. She thought she had lost her mind because there was no basis for her fears. Her husband was a careful, level-headed driver. Then she remembered that when she was a child, her father drove like a maniac and her mother pretended that everything was fine. She covered up her real feelings. Had her mother admitted her fears, had they been able to talk about it, there would have been no duplicity and the woman wouldn't have felt she was losing her mind.

Oh, all the things that come to light after many years of therapy! I have a woman coming to see me quite regularly. She has been coming for over 10 years. Recently, we spoke about how her father used her sexually, and it took her quite a while to start remembering it. Her relationships didn't work out and she has been living on her own for a long time. She could never really have enjoyable sex because the memories of forced sex with her father always disturbed her. So, she considered seeing a sex therapist who had sex with traumatised women in a slow, gentle, non-threatening way. It wasn't an easy decision but eventually she took the plunge. She's been meeting him regularly for over a year now. She is finding it difficult not to fall in love with him. But she realised something I would have never thought of: she has several men in her life whom she pays for service. A physiotherapist, the sex therapist, a trainer, me and another therapist. She spends a lot of money on these men and suddenly this became clear to her. I was pondering how much she would have had to pay to her father so he wouldn't have sexually abused her.

She remembered that money was the only thing her father loved more than sex. You pay a therapist, so they don't have desires, and this woman realised that she is spending a lot of money on feeling safe. She can't conceive of any other kind of relationship. She is perhaps punishing herself. We have gone through and around this a thousand times but she still thinks that she should have said no to her father and that she was somehow his accomplice. Deep down, she can't accept that the responsibility belongs to her father a hundred percent. Perhaps it's less frightening to accept that she was bad than to accept that she was utterly powerless and unprotected. If it takes this long with this very intelligent woman until reason prevails over a false sense of responsibility, then it must create major problems for others too. This, of course, also includes the fact that she isn't able to have the full experience that therapy could be. As long as she is convinced that the only reason men in her life don't hurt her is because she gives them money, she will annihilate the experience of being loved. She will think the only reason I don't hurt her is because she is paying me, because I'm a professional. I don't hurt her out of fear of consequences, not out of caring for her. Is she taking revenge? Is she punishing herself and me? Mourning eludes her. Every man turns into her father, although the man who happened to be her father was an evil, devious, dumb-ass prick. The stork could have tossed her into a family where the father would have loved and protected her. It's hard for her to realise it's not her fault, it's just bad luck. It's very painful to think of what happened as being hit by a drunk driver, a stupid accident, nothing personal. She lives as if she were poor, she doesn't want to grow up and she is always playing the game of a little child who is being taken advantage of. She is constantly complaining that her therapists are exploiting her, but at least not sexually, only financially. She thinks that when we renovated our house, she had paid for that, and when her sex therapist went to the Bahamas with his girlfriend, they paid for the holiday with the money she gave him. Instead of nourishing herself with wild adventures, she gives away her resources to these safe professionals. Why is she afraid of her freedom? Could she stop the whole thing and live her own experiences without her therapists? Why does she not do that? The reason, I think, is because, perhaps unconsciously, she takes some secret pleasure in having control; there is some hidden thrill in it for her. *Jouissance* and not *plaisir*.[33] She chooses the hidden delight and not the open pleasure. She replays the disaster again and again; how can she ever trust, hope or relax again, after such betrayal? People follow and repeat this pattern because it makes us feel in control of the situation. We can recreate the problem or the trauma. When it first happened, it was like a bolt of lightning out of the blue, but by repeating the pattern, we feel we have mastered it and prefer to hurt ourselves rather than open up to new uncertainties. Of course, it is easy to say all of the above, but very difficult to discuss it with her without the danger of blaming her, of blaming the victim. I feel nothing but a deep sadness that the impact of her father's predation is so very difficult to recover from.

Traditional Freudianism only promises that, by the end of psychotherapy, the patient will have an increased capacity for suffering. According to this school of thought, this is the only thing that can be promised. In other words, suffering doesn't decrease, but one doesn't have to worry that their suffering will be greater than what they can tolerate. Freud would have considered it too ambitious to try to increase freedom. I often have the experience that my patients are freer after therapy than when they first started seeing me. One of the most important things a therapist can do is encourage their patient. The crucial question is not "why?" but "why not?". Georges Devereux,[34] a Hungarian-born anthropologist and psychoanalyst, working in France, stated that he had realised one has to fight for one's freedom until the end of one's life, until the grave. One cannot secure freedom once and for all because someone will always come and try, willy-nilly, to take it away, so we must always be ready to fight for it. This made him feel despondent, at first. He didn't even want to continue living. It all seemed too exhausting. He disappeared for a year, didn't talk to anyone, and then he returned to life in a jolly mood and decided to enjoy the constant readiness to fight for freedom. What's more, he couldn't wait for someone to try to take away his freedom and give him a chance to fight for it, like Clint Eastwood, in the 1983 film *Sudden Impact*, saying, "Go ahead, make my day!" Devereux grew to love the fight so much that if someone offered to fight in his place, he wouldn't allow it, just as, he said, he wouldn't allow someone other than himself to sleep with his wife. A therapist can't encourage more freedom in their patient than what they have managed to obtain for themselves. If the patient is freer than the therapist, then the therapist ought to pay them. People don't do what you tell them to do but what they see you do. Relationships in society, at present, are no better and no worse than they have ever been. One has always had to fight for freedom. The Inquisition used to torture those who dared to say freely what they thought, despite knowing full well that they would be impaled on the stake, quartered, or pulled apart by horses. There is nothing new under the sun.

"Shall we be slaves or men set free?"[35] Free of course. You must be crazy to say anything else. But what kind of choice is that, really? What is slavery and what is freedom? We can become slaves at any given moment even if others consider us free. At other times, we can be free even if others consider us slaves. A deeply cherished little girl becomes a tormented orphaned slave the moment her father touches her sexually. A prisoner serving countless years turns into a king as he becomes absorbed in playing the title role of a stage show. The little girl loses her freedom because she is not supposed to talk about what is important and because she is afraid that no one will take her seriously and no one will protect her. Her captivity is from the words being constrained and locked in; the prisoner's curious liberation comes from the momentary freedom of words, thoughts and emotions, from being able to play their roles, feeling safe and unashamed in the here and now. The father wants to take advantage of his daughter; he has power over her, that's how the child becomes a slave. At the end of the day, abusers dare abuse their victims because they think they have worked out a way they can do it without consequences or punishment. The glint in the eye of the abuser is the delight in getting away with it. This calculation gives strength and framework to the power. But every framework can be questioned. In the '60s, many young people from the north travelled to the southern states of the US to encourage African Americans to travel to the northern states where human rights were respected, where they could live in safety, and where there was much more freedom. This was about power: go to the place where you have the power to change things. Nobody can smuggle power into the prison. The prisoners are divested of their power by the justice system. That's the price they pay for their crimes. But we can take love into the prison: love free from all shades of sentimentality, love that gives a sense of security, and then the prisoners can play in a place that we never thought could become a playground.

In a letter to a young therapist, Gregory Bateson writes about free will. It was the first time in the professional career of this young therapist that one of his patients committed suicide and he was in anguish about how the patient would still be alive if he had done or said things differently, or if he had not done or said things. To console him, Bateson attempted to prove to him that he couldn't have been the cause of the patient's death. Either everyone has free will or nobody has it. It is not possible that some people have free will while others don't. Consequently, there are two possibilities in this specific case: if there's no free will, if everything is predetermined, then both the patient's actions and the therapist's behaviour are preordained. If this is the case, there is no leeway, no opportunity to make decisions, no responsibility, and therefore no problem. The second possibility is that free will exists. If this is the case, the therapist could have said and done things differently but the actions of the patient would also not be predetermined, so they could have reacted in countless ways to the therapist's words and actions. Killing themself was only one of a thousand different options, but this was what they chose.[36]

I often use this logic when working with couples. If one of them looks at the other and says, "If you leave me, I'll kill myself," I find it crucial to state immediately in front of both of them that they are both free. They are free to leave each other. We have to be clear that, if this were not the case, they couldn't be free to be together either. One of them leaving the other and the other making threats of suicide is not a direct consequence of abandonment. We know, as Bateson argues, that the abandoned spouse could react in a thousand different ways and suicide is only one of these options. But the responsibility for this choice belongs entirely to the person who makes it. If the deserted party knows that the person abandoning them won't torment themself over them, this knowledge will take the wind out of their sails because they obviously won't be able to take revenge in this way.

In his book *Insomnia*, Henry Miller writes about how hellishly difficult it is to really love someone. The author is in his seventies and lives with his love, a gorgeous young Asian chanteuse. Every night, around four in the morning, the girl comes home from the bar where she sings, and every night, the author waits up for her, burning in the hellish torments of jealousy. Miller is in anguish but he knows that the moment he tries to restrict the freedom of the woman even slightly, he will lose her. Every word of the book is squeezed from the torment suffered while waiting for her.

Practically up until his death, Sartre insisted that love didn't actually exist and talking about love was just a trick. Human relationships aren't based on love but on power, because if I can make someone believe they love me, it is easy to take advantage of them or dominate them. Just before his death, however, Sartre wrote with a little contrition that, ultimately, he did understand, he did recognise the existence of love.[37] So, why did he not see love before, why did he not recognise the obvious? Because he wasn't interested. Just like a pickpocket who was introduced to Buddha only saw Buddha's pockets, Sartre similarly interpreted every example of love's manifestation as a power game. His understanding eventually came from connecting freedom and love. His new realization – knowing that someone loves you when you feel freer in their company than on your own – was a total paradigm shift in his interpretation of human relationships.

Levinas, on the other hand, maintains that I can only be completely free when I am on my own because the very moment another person's face turns towards me, a sense of responsibility emerges in me. If more people turn towards me, I have to face the issues of justice and fairness. According to Levinas, the "Thou shall not kill!" commandment is written on the face of the other.[38] The impulse to do everything I can for the other and to give them my everything if they need it is not really a free choice, it is an atavistic, anarchic commandment. The Winnicottian "good enough mother" is a basic example of this conviction. The mother will make sacrifices without thinking and she will give her life for the life or well-being of her child.[39] This is why I call this ethics *maternal ethics*. This instinct can be released, and it can be found if we deeply accept and envision everyone alive as our child while also thinking of ourselves as everyone's child. So, just as a baby could, I can rely on others' benevolence and not just on them expecting my kindness. In this context, egoistic freedom drives us towards evil because it incites rebellion against a deep inner impulse. Lucifer refused to serve; life was not sacred to him.

All this clearly demonstrates that we can talk about freedom within the ego or beyond the ego. "What do I do when I don't know what to do?" is a fundamental question for all of us. The ego always wants to do something. It would feel ashamed if it had to admit that it didn't know what to do. The ego's freedom is that it can do anything but this stubbornness can create a lot of damage. In my opinion, "nothing" is the best answer to the above question. You need to wait until the situation moves you. If this is true, then freedom should be understood as it is in the Bible: "Thy will be done."[40] It is good to be free to do nothing and to be free to give myself over to the will of the situation.

If we closely examine the phenomenology of sex, we come to the same conclusion. If sex were under the control of the ego, the cock would be a muscle and men could move it like a finger. I don't think an individual actually possesses sexuality. Real sexuality emerges between people. In normal circumstances, the cock becomes erect in the erotic space between two (or more) people, as the lovers are together in that space. Guy de Maupassant was boasting to Flaubert, and apparently he demonstrated that he could make his cock erect whenever he wanted; he just counted to three and that was that.[41] I think this is a brilliant exhibition for a circus show but it is nothing compared to the opportunity in sex to give ourselves to the situation, to the other person, and to a reality beyond the ego. Nowadays, modern sexology is almost totally based on supporting the ego. When a man is labelled impotent in a relationship, medical science's response is to insert a plastic rod into his penis, to administer an injection before making love or to install a pump in his scrotum. In my practice, sometimes there seems to be a simpler solution, which is to bring out into the open that the spouses haven't been attracted to each other for a long time. Quite often, the very moment a man is free to look for a partner who is attractive to him, his impotence is cured. And of course, the same applies to women's ability to swell and moisten their vulvas and to orgasm.

It is worth saying a few words about the apparent antithesis of freedom: addiction. In every kind of addiction, from heroin and alcohol to sex, the basic problem is that the person is not able or doesn't want to stop. Again, the real question is whether one is free or whether their actions are predetermined. Wanting to want something is not the same as wanting it. In our culture, or rather in the way we use language, and perhaps both, it is permitted to say: "I want to want something, but unfortunately, I cannot do it, I am not able to want it. I am trying, I am endeavouring, but it is not happening." My purpose in saying this is to make the other person think that I am a good person who is simply weak or ill. In my opinion, we get much closer to reality if we pronounce such a "good but weak" person to be simply "bad". Once we are clear on this, we can respect the other person's freedom and we won't pretend that they need treatment. By "bad" I don't mean, of course, some character flaw or a definition of their personality. I use it as an adjective to describe the person who is doing something destructive in that given moment. Even if I do bad things often and for a long time, I will still always have a free choice. I can always turn back and never do anything bad ever again. There is no need for atonement. The gods will forgive me. So, I don't have to feel ashamed of myself but it is good to feel guilty for my actions. Shame would kill me but guilt can be relieved because I can always rectify what I have done. I can always set things right. Every moment is critical and every moment only ever happens once. We can quit any habit, including any addiction, at any moment. Or maybe, to put it in a different way, we can wake up. Habits and addictions are illusions, dreams. The reality is complete freedom.

It is never easy to give up our habits. It is possible, but not easy. Among other goals, all forms of meditation also aim to free us from automatic habitual patterns to let us hear the echoes of the heart. This is what meditation gives us the tools for. To achieve this, it is crucial to slow down and pay attention to what is happening, to what we are doing. Everyone has the experience that if we are driving too fast on the highway, we won't even notice possible exits. The things we don't notice cease to be opportunities, so we lose our freedom because of our speed. Unfortunately, just understanding that I am a slave to my habits is not enough to get rid of them. Even when I can clearly see the exit coming up, when I can see the chance to leave the routine motorway and turn off onto an unknown road, it is still surprisingly difficult to make this decision. I need courage and the full force of my willpower to leave the habitual direction. Going against the grain is difficult but possible. Masters of meditation all teach us that the practitioner should treat themself gently. Don't despair if you don't always succeed in what you want to do. For example, when we count our breaths – out, in: *one*, out, in: *two*, and so on to ten – then notice we lost count, got distracted by an unexpected train of thought and forgot to count, there's no problem. No matter how long we got distracted for, we can just gently return to "one".

In families without a strong will, pressure or defined direction children have to follow, youngsters grow up to be spontaneous, honest and authentic. The greater the family pressure, the more children forget what they want. They lose their own freedom because all their time is taken up by reacting to others' will. So, they either obey and perform what's expected of them, comply, or they rebel and resist. Neither compliance nor rebellion are authentic. But the above-mentioned family is a rare bird. Most people, including me, can only find the road to being authentic by spending an extraordinary amount of time in a "vacuum", in let's say therapy and/or meditation, where one is shielded from other people's opinions, desires and wishes, and can finally pay attention to one's own heart. "Listen to the silence of your own heart!" as Mother Teresa taught. But we have neglected our hearts for years, so why would it speak to us now, just because we are suddenly paying attention? We have to reassure our heart that from now on, we will never neglect it again and then, miracle of miracles, it just might start speaking.

I was living on the fourth floor of a house in Kis Rókus street, in Buda, with my mother, and whenever it started snowing, I had to wear galoshes. My mother wouldn't even let me out the door without them. And I hated galoshes. I always took them off on the second floor, hid them and then put them on again on my way back home. So, my mother continued to believe that I was her obedient, good little boy. When I was 18, living on my own in Toronto, I quite often got home with my shoes and socks soaked through if the weather was wet or there was big snow outside. I started pondering this: would it be an admission of my mother being right, would I betray myself, if I started wearing galoshes? It wasn't easy to unravel whether I could want to wear galoshes authentically, out of my own free will, despite the fact that that's what my mother would want. Eventually, I started wearing galoshes because I realised that one can be authentic even if they do what their mother would have wanted. These galoshes are not those galoshes.

Another story to illustrate how difficult this question is: My father and mother divorced when I was five. I lived with my mother and visited my father once a week. When I was seven, during one of my visits, my father ceremoniously handed me some money and said that, from then on, I would get weekly pocket money. On my way home, I happily bought myself a few things and, on the corner, before turning onto our street, I stopped at the florist. I bought my mother a bouquet of flowers and proudly gave it to her. Later, I heard her boasting to her friend on the phone that her son bought her flowers from his first pocket money. The next week, I bought a model plane kit with my money and spent my last pennies on glue. As soon as I got home, I started building the plane. I soon noticed there was a heavy, tense atmosphere in the flat. My mother went about her chores fuming. I asked her what was wrong. "Where are my flowers?" she snapped. I was ashamed because my negligence proved how selfish I was. After that, I often stopped at the florist, but I could never ever buy her flowers again spontaneously, with a good heart.

In my practice, all the people who are most desperate, who are suffering from the most serious kind of depression, want to commit suicide because they can't fathom how to break free from the roles they have been chronically stuck in since childhood. A woman told me that she had to play the role of a nice little girl for her parents at home, in school she had to play the role of a good pupil, and then she became her husband's good wife. She told her husband several times that she didn't want children, and still, she gave birth to two kids. She first attempted suicide after the birth of her second child. On top of all her other roles, now she would have to play the role of a good mother as well. This thought proved too much to bear.

It takes a lot of courage and practice to actually feel free. Remember what I told you about Georges Devereux? You cannot avoid always being ready for a battle and anticipating an aggressor. One who doesn't want to fight for their freedom cannot enjoy their life.

There are two kinds of learning. We easily understand the things we shouldn't do because learning avoidance is one-trial learning. For example, we quickly learn not to put our hand in the fire; it is enough to try only once. But learning to play the piano is not as simple. You have to practise ten thousand hours to be able to play well. I am 80, yet I still practise being courageous, loving, and just listening.

R.D. Laing's 12 Recommended Books:

1. Anonymous: *The Cloud of Unknowing*
2. Pseudo-Dionysius the Areopagite: *Mystical Theology* and *The Celestial Hierarchy*
3. Pascal, Blaise: *Pensées*
4. Montaigne, Michel de: *"On Experience" (essay)*
5. Plato: *Republic*
6. Plato: *Phaedrus*
7. Plato: *Parmenides*
8. Pre-Socratic fragments, especially Heraclitus
9. Kierkegaard, Søren: *The Sickness unto Death* *[Sygdommen til Deden]*
10. Kierkegaard, Søren: *Either/Or [Enten-Eller]*
11. Shestov, Lev: *In Job's Balances*
12. Bible: Ecclesiastes; St John's Gospel

Notes

EPIGRAPHS

1 Giorgio Agamben. (2007). *Profanations* (J. Fort, Trans.). Zone Books, New York.

2 John Fowles. (1964). *The Aristos: A Self-Portrait in Ideas*. Little, Brown and Company, Boston.

INTRODUCTION

1 Francis Huxley (1923–2016) was a British botanist, anthropologist and writer, whom Feldmár met and befriended in London, England. Huxley was close friends with Laing and acted as Director of Studies at Laing's Philadelphia Association (PA). Leon Redler (b 1936) is a British psychiatrist, psychotherapist and teacher, whom Feldmár also met in London. Redler was a fellow student and member of the PA and also worked in one of the shelters they ran. Redler continues, today, to teach for the PA. David Bakan (1921–2004) was an American psychologist, historian, philosopher and scholar who attempted to find the roots of psychology in Jewish mysticism and the Kabbalah. For further information, please see his Encyclopedia Britannica entry: https://www.britannica.com/ biography/ David-Bakan. His wife, Mildred Bakan (1922–2010), was one of the first female philosophy academics in Canada. She taught and wrote in the areas of philosophy and social sciences, was a community activist and political scholar. For more information, please see the Mildred Bakan fonds at the York University Library: https://atom.library.yorku.ca /index.php/mildred-bakan-fonds.

2 David Abram (b 1957) is a philosopher, ecologist, magician, and founder of Alliance for Wild Ethics. For more information about his work, please

see his book, *The Spell of the Sensuous: Perception and Language in a More-than-Human World* (1996. Random House, New York.), and his bio on the Wild Ethics website: https://wildethics.org/alliance-members/abram/.

3   Zalman Schachter-Shalomi (1924–2014), commonly known as Reb Zalman, was a radical rabbi, a mystic, a founder of the Jewish Renewal and the inventor of ecumenical dialogue, which promoted the unity of all Christian religions. For further information, please see this biography: https://www.colorado.edu/post-holocaustamericanjudaismcollections/home/biography-zalman-schachter-shalomi.

4   The Arrow Cross was a far-right Hungarian party led by Ferenc Szálasi that formed a government in Hungary in 1944, known as the Government of National Unity.

5   Emmanuel Levinas (1906–1995) was a French philosopher of Lithuanian Jewish descent. His main areas of interest were phenomenology, ethics, ontology and Judaism. Levinas writes about the "stranger" in both *Totality and Infinity* (1969. Duquesne UP, Pittsburgh.) and later, more expansively, in *Otherwise than Being or Beyond Essence* (1981. Duquesne UP, Pittsburgh.).

6   Martin Buber was a philosopher, scholar, and worked heavily with Hasidic Lore and Judaism. He is most well known for his work on dialogue within existentialism, as laid out in his book, *I and Thou* (1970. Charles Scribner's Sons, New York.).

7   Mishnah: Pirkei Avot - Ethics of the Fathers, 1:14.

8   R.D. Laing and his colleagues, mentioned above, founded the Philadelphia Association in 1965 to provide shelter for those who would have otherwise been committed to mental asylums. Later, they also founded a school for teaching psychotherapy and milieu therapy in therapy communities. For further information, please see the PA website: https://www. philadelphia-association.com/.

RUPTURES

[1] "József Attila: The Seventh One (*A hetedik* in English)". (G. Gyukics and M. Castro, Trans.). *Babelmatrix: Babel Web Anthology – the Multilingual Literature Portal.* https://www.babelmatrix.org/works/hu/J%C3%B3zsef_Attila-1905/A_hetedik/en/54608-The_Seventh_One.

[2] Joseph Brodsky (1940–1996) was a Russian poet, exiled in 1972. He settled in the USA, won a Nobel Prize for literature and gave three different university commencement addresses. Feldmár's paraphrase, here, is from Brodsky's 1984 Commencement Address at Williams College, in Massachusetts. For the full text, please see https://www.nybooks.com/articles/1984/08/16/a-commencement-address/.

[3] Joan Halifax (b 1942), also known as Roshi Joan, is the founder of the Upaya Zen Center in Santa Fé, New Mexico. One of her prominent teachers was Roshi Berni Glassman, an American Zen Buddhist and founder of the Zen Peacemakers. Halifax has studied anthropology, psychology and shamanism, as well as Buddhism and certain radical practices in all these disciplines. She has worked with Joseph Campbell and Stanislav Grof, and published eight books since 1968, including *The Human Encounter with Death*, which she co-authored with Grof and was published in 1977 by E.P. Dutton in Boston. For more information about Roshi Joan, please see her bio: https://www.upaya.org/about/roshi/.

[4] Gregory Bateson (1904–1980) was an anthropologist, social scientist, philosopher and linguist. His work and scholarship crossed into many other disciplines, including psychology. His theory called the "double bind" was important because it laid out a specific kind of environment that could, potentially, produce a schizophrenic individual. Bateson and his colleagues published an article about it, "Toward a Theory of Schizophrenia", in *Behavioral Science* in 1956 (1(4): 251–254).

⁵ Thomas Szász (1920–2012) was a Hungarian-born American psychologist and psychiatrist, perhaps best known for his anti-psychiatric stance. For more about Szász's idea that mental illness does not exist, see his book *The Myth of Mental Illness: Foundations of a Theory of Personal Conduct* (1961. Harper, New York.).

⁶ George Ivanovitch Gurdjieff (1866–1949) was a Russian philosopher, mystic and spiritual teacher, and has been hailed as one of the most important spiritual teachers of the 20th century. One of his early students, P.D. Ouspensky, carried on Gurdjieff's teaching and wrote about all of it in *In Search of the Miraculous: Fragments of an Unknown Teaching*, published in 1949 by Harcourt Brace, California. The book lays out Gurdjieff's methods more than any other.

⁷ Phyllis Chesler (b 1940) is an author, psychotherapist, professor emeritus, feminist leader, community organiser and scholar of the global rise of antisemitism. For more information about Chesler and her work, please see her website: https://phyllis-chesler.com/.

⁸ Latin: first among equals.

⁹ Stanislav Grof (b 1931) is a Czech-born radical and psychedelic psychiatrist known for his life-long study of altered states of consciousness and LSD psychotherapy, and as one of the founders of transpersonal psychology. For further information, please see the bio on his website, http://www.stangrof.com/.

¹⁰ The books Feldmár received are the *Tractatus Logico-Philosophicus* (1922) by Ludwig Wittgenstein and *Gravity and Grace* (1947) by Simone Weil.

ORIGINS

¹ David Cooper, a South African psychiatrist, was one of the founders of the Philadelphia Association, along with Laing. He was important in the anti-psychiatry movement and is said to have coined that term. For more

information, please see his books *Psychiatry and Anti-Psychiatry* (1967, Tavistock) and *The Language of Madness* (1978, Allen Lane).

[2] The skeptics were one of the three branches of ancient Hellenistic Greek philosophy, along with the Stoics and the Epicureans. There were academic skeptics and Pyrrhonian skeptics, and we are interested in the latter here. Their main objectives were to question certainty and suspend judgement. According to John Heaton, they "all practised philosophy as a way of addressing and alleviating the most painful problems of human life." In other words, these philosophers behaved like therapists. Please see John M. Heaton (1997) "Pyrrhonian Scepticism: A Therapeutic Phenomenology. *Journal of the British Society for Phenomenology*, 28:1, 80-96.

[3] John Heaton. (2010). *The Talking Cure: Wittgenstein's Therapeutic Method for Psychotherapy*. Palgrave Macmillan, London. The connection here is that Wittgenstein was, according to Heaton, as against dogmatics as the Skeptics were. The Greek word *skepsis* means "investigation", something Wittgenstein was extremely interested in. This connects strongly with Laing, who thought psychotherapy was an "inquiry".

[4] Francis Huxley passed away on October 29, 2016, in Santa Fé, NM, USA.

JOURNAL ENTRIES 1974–75, LONDON

[1] *Voices* is a journal, published three times a year by the American Academy of Psychotherapists. From their website: "It focuses on the personal struggles and growth of therapists and the influences of therapists on the process of psychotherapy." For more information, please see https://www.aapweb.net/voices.html.

[2] T.S. Eliot. (1931). "Preface" to *Transit of Venus: Poems by Harry Crosby*. Black Sun Press, Paris.

[3] Wilfred R. Bion (1897-1979) was an influential British psychoanalyst who was president of the British Psychoanalytical Society from 1962 to 1965.

335

For more information on his work with groups and communities, please see his book, *Experiences in Groups: and Other Papers* (1961. Tavistock, London).

4   Benjamin Disraeli (1804–1881), 1st Earl of Beaconsfield, was the prime minister of the United Kingdom twice and was the Conservative Party leader. He was also a novelist. This quote is widely attributed to him; however, no source has been found.

5   In mathematics, a lemma is a proven proposition which is used as a stepping stone to more significant results. In other words, it is a subsidiary or intermediate theorem in an argument or proof.

6   Stanley Keleman (1931–2018) was an American writer and therapist, who was one of the leaders of the body psychotherapy movement. For more on his thoughts about death, please see his book *Living your Dying* (1975. Random House, New York.).

7   William Blake (1757–1827) was an English poet, mystic, artist, and visionary, who is hailed as one of the most important figures of the Romantic era. Feldmár's paraphrase here is from Blake's *Songs of Innocence and of Experience* (1789), particularly from the second part, "Songs of Experience".

8   In actual fact, both the words "speculate" and "speculum" come from the Latin *speculari*, meaning "to observe", which comes from *specer* "to look at", based on both Walter W. Skeat's 1884 *Concise Dictionary of English Etymology*, republished by Wordsworth in 2007, and the Online Etymology Dictionary, etymonline.com.) "Speculum", while not etymologically related to the word "mirror", is a word that means an instrument used for observing, a looking glass, or a mirror. "Mirror", on the other hand, comes from a variant of the Latin *mirari*, meaning "to wonder at, admire", and is where we get the English word "miracle".

9   The information given here, about the word "guilt" is incorrect, based on both Skeat and the Online Etymology Dictionary. Nowhere do these

mention any connection to the Latin *torquere* or turning or twisting in any way. However, the Online Etymology Dictionary does say its origin is unknown. "Torment", "torture", and "distort", are words that come directly from *torquere*. "Guilt" is from Old/Middle English *gylt*, meaning "crime, sin and/or fine, to pay a debt". It is that source that is of unknown origin.

10 D.W. Winnicott (1896–1971) was an English paediatrician and psychoanalyst, whose theories took a departure from the Freudian perspective. Winnicott focussed on early childhood, child–parent relationships, object relations, and the importance of play in development. For more information about what Feldmár says here, see Winnicott's paper, "Hate in the Counter-Transference" (1949. *The International Journal of Psychoanalysis*, 30, 69–74) and his book Through Paediatrics to Psychoanalysis, first published in 1958 by Basic Books in New York.

11 Medard Boss (1903–1990) was a Swiss psychoanalyst and psychiatrist who worked elements of existentialism and phenomenology into his understanding and theories of psychoanalysis, developing a twenty-year-long friendship with Heidegger and inventing his own form of Daseinsanalysis. For more information, please see Boss's book, *Existential Foundations of Medicine and Psychology*, originally published in 1977 by Jason Aronson in Maryland.

12 John C. Lilly (1915–2001) was a neuroscientist, psychoanalyst, and counter-cultural explorer of human consciousness with Timothy Leary and others. His first two books, both published in the 1960s, are about dolphins and launched the global interest and study of ocean mammals. For more information about Lilly and his work, please visit https://www.johnclilly.com/.

13 Francis Huxley. (1956). *Affable Savages: An Anthropologist Among the Urubu Indians of Brazil*. Hart-Davis, London.

[14] John Bowlby (1907–1990) was a British psychotherapist who did pioneering work in attachment theory and wrote *Separation: Anxiety and Anger*, published in 1973 by Basic Books, New York.

[15] Arica is a human-potential movement group founded in 1968 by Bolivian-born philosopher Oscar Ichazo (b 1931). The Arica school was described in 1973, by Ramparts magazine, as "A body of techniques for cosmic consciousness-raising and an ideology to relate to the world in an awakened way." Ichazo is considered the father of the Enneagram of Personality. For more information, please see https://www.arica.org/.

[16] B.K.S. Iyengar (1918–2014), yoga teacher, started teaching in 1936, at the age of 18, in Pune, India. In 1973, he founded the world-famous Ramamani Iyengar Memorial Yoga Institute. He is the author of many books; his first, *Light on Yoga*, is considered a classic today. His teaching is firmly based on Patanjali's ancient yoga sutras.

[17] Rolfing is a massage therapy system developed in 1971 by Ida Pauline Rolf at her Rolf Institute of Structural Integration (RISI).

[18] Masud Khan (1924–1989) was a Pakistani-British psychoanalyst who trained and apprenticed under D.W. Winnicott and Anna Freud. His life and work were very controversial, and he made significant contributions to the psychoanalytic field. For more about his work on perversion, please see his books *The Privacy of the Self* (1974) and *Alienation in Perversions* (1979), both originally published by The Hogarth Press, London.

[19] Otto Rank (1884–1939) was an Austrian psychoanalyst and teacher. He was a close colleague and protégé of Freud's for at least 20 years. Rank was a pioneer in extending psychoanalytic work to include legends and myths. Carl Jung was influenced by him, as was Carl Rogers. His book *The Trauma of Birth*, was originally published, as *Das Trauma der Geburt*, in 1924, by Internationaler Psychoanalytischer Verlag. The first English translation came out in 1929 from Kegan Paul, Trench, Trubner and Co. in London.

[20] "Catullus 85" is a poem written by the Roman poet Gaius Valerius Catullus to his lover. Catullus is thought to have lived from around 84 BC to about 54 BC. Translator unknown.

[21] Feldmár was reading D.W. Winnicott's book *The Child, The Family and the Outside World*, which was originally published in 1964 by Penguin Books in Harmondsworth, UK. The reference here comes from chapter 12 of that book.

[22] Konstantin Sergeyevich Stanislavski (1863–1938) was a Russian actor and director with groundbreaking achievements in actor-training and theory. He was one of the founders of the Moscow Art Theatre and developed a system for training actors that, among other things, was meant to activate the will. For more information, please see his books *An Actor's Work: A Student's Diary* (1938) and *An Actor's Work on a Role* (1957).

[23] An old Scots word from Gaelic, and later Scottish, that means a traditional gathering with music, singing, and storytelling.

[24] Francis J. Mott (1901–1990) was a British publisher and intellectual who developed his psychological ideas and theories of the self while spending much time in Canada and the USA. Two major books of his, available today from Starwalker Press, are The Nature of the Self (1959. Allen Wingate, London.) and *Mythology of the Prenatal Life* (1960. The Integration Publishing Company, UK.), both published in the UK. For more information on Mott, please see https://www.starwalkerpress.com/MottBio.htm.

[25] The morula is the small mass of divided cells created by the initial fertilisation of the ovum, from which the blastula forms. A blastula is defined as an early metazoan embryo typically having the form of a hollow fluid-filled rounded cavity bounded by a single layer of cells. It is the result of repeated cell division, the morula, and is the earliest form of an embryo possible.

[26] Victor Tausk (1879–1919) was an Austrian psychoanalyst who was a student and colleague of Freud's. During the First World War, he was a

medic and those experiences influenced his psychoanalytic work, which focussed on psychosis and personality. His most famous paper, "On the Origin of the 'Influencing Machine' in Schizophrenia", was written and published in 1919, just months before Tausk committed suicide. Nándor Fodor (1895–1964) was a Hungarian-born British and American psychoanalyst, parapsychologist, and journalist. His work, especially his 1949 book *The Search for the Beloved: A Clinical Investigation of the Trauma of Birth and Pre-Natal Conditioning*, published by Hermitage Press in New Jersey, exerted influence in the burgeoning field of prenatal psychology.

[27] Grof developed a map of the psyche, which he believes is partly formed during what he considers the four stages of birth. He called these stages basic perinatal matrixes, or BPMs. BPM II is called "cosmic engulfment and no exit". For more information, please see Grof's book *The Adventure of Self-Discovery. Dimensions of Consciousness and New Perspectives in Psychotherapy and Inner Exploration*, published in 1988 by SUNY Press, for more information.

[28] D.W. Winnicott. (1965). *The Maturational Processes and the Facilitating Environment: Studies in the Theory of Emotional Development*. Karnac Books, London.

[29] Latin: mode of operating. It means the way something works, or how one works and/or functions.

[30] Oliver Sacks (1933–2015) was a naturalist, a writer and a medical doctor who specialised in neurology. It is often said that he regarded the human brain as the most interesting thing in the universe. One of his books, Awakenings, published in 1973 by Duckworth & Co., London, was later used as the basis for a movie of the same name that came out in 1990, starring Robin Williams and Robert De Niro. He was an award-winning author, writing almost exclusively about his patient's neurological case histories and his own unusual experiences due to his neurological condition.

[31] Victoria Sweet is a physician, author and advocate of slow medicine. For more information about her and the slow medicine movement, please see https://www.victoriasweet.com/.

[32] Francis Huxley was able to read French, and is referring here to material from the original 1972 French publication of *Anti-Oedipus, L'anti-Œdipe,* by Gilles Deleuze and Félix Guattari.

[33] The Palo Alto Mental Research Institute was founded in 1958 by Don D. Jackson and was instrumental in starting both brief and family therapy within the general field of psychotherapy. Jackson was a member of Gregory Bateson's "Project", which was a collaboration of schizophrenia researchers that ran from 1953 to 1963. They worked with Jackson as medical director and Gregory Bateson as theoretical director.

[34] Latin: a faulty or vicious cycle.

[35] Carl Jung (1875–1961) was a Swiss psychologist and psychoanalyst, credited with founding analytic psychology. He was a friend and colleague of Freud's initially, but then they went their separate ways. He is known for delineating extraverted and inverted character types, coming up with the notion of the collective unconscious (which includes all his dream interpretation work), and creating archetypes. Feldmár was reading from Jung's then-unpublished lectures from 1936 and '37, most likely shared with him by Haya Oakley. These lectures were later published, most recently by Princeton University Press in 2019 as *Dream Symbols of the Individuation Process: Notes of C. G. Jung's Seminars on Wolfgang Pauli's Dreams.*

[36] Neogenesis is a biological term that means regeneration, new or renewed formation, usually of tissue.

[37] Niccolò Machiavelli (1469–1527) was an Italian political philosopher, a statesman and an author. The source for this, the book Feldmár is referring to, is *The Prince* (1532).

[38] Judith Herman (b 1942) is an American psychologist, researcher, teacher

and author. She has, throughout her career, focused on trauma, both surviving it and recovering from it, including incest. Feldmár is referring to information from her book *Trauma and Recovery*, published in 1992 by Basic Books in New York.

[39] *Did You Used to Be R.D. Laing?* (1989). Directed by Thomas Shandel and Kirk Tougas. The full documentary is available on YouTube, at https://www.youtube.com/watch?v=86t5GWB5qRY.

[40] ECT stands for electroconvulsive therapy, which is the newer term for electroshock therapy.

[41] Erik H. Erikson. (1964). *Insight and Responsibility: Lectures on the Ethical Implications of Psychoanalytic Insight*. W.W. Norton & Co., New York.

[42] D.W. Winnicott. (1971). *Therapeutic Consultations in Child Psychiatry* Hogarth Press, London.

[43] "Metanoia", from Greek, is a combination of *meta*, which means "change", and *noein*, which means "mental perception". In English, it usually refers to a spiritual conversion. It can also simply refer to a personal transformation.

[44] "Nobody knows the trouble I've seen" is an old African-American spiritual song, originating from the period of slavery. It was first recorded in the 1867 book *Slave Songs of the United States*, publisher unknown. It has since been covered by many musicians, including Louis Armstrong, on his 1958 album *Louis and the Good Book*.

[45] Ram Dass (1931–2019), born Richard Alpert, was a spiritual guide, yoga teacher, psychologist, psychedelic researcher and author. His work, including his most famous book, *Be Here Now* (1971. Lama Foundation, New Mexico), was integral to bringing multiple Eastern spiritual forms to the West. For more information about him, his life, and his work, please see https://www.ramdass.org/ about-ram-dass/.

[46] Rainer Maria Rilke (1875–1926) was an Austrian poet and literary artist. He is widely considered one of the most lyrically intense German-language

poets. His work is often considered mystical and is also quite existential. His best-known works include *The Duino Elegies* (1923) and *Letters to a Young Poet* (1929).

47   Robert W. Firestone (b 1930) is an American psychologist, writer, and artist. His work, although developed separately from Laing's, was very similar, as this quote from the "About" section of Firestone's website shows: his work "focused on the concept that defenses formed by individuals early in life tend to impede the individuation process, often impair their ability to sustain intimate adult relationships, and can have a damaging effect on their children." For more information, please see https://www.drrobertwfirestone.com/ biography. Firestone's approach to working with and treating patients labelled "schizophrenic", was aligned more with Laing's than with the traditional medical models. He was an adept sailor, and it was his yacht they were on.

48   See note 41, above, about the Erikson source.

49   Gaston Bachelard (1884–1962) wrote and published *La psychanalyse du feu* (1938), which was translated and published as *The Psychoanalysis of Fire* in 1964; *L'eau et les rêves* (1942), which was translated and published as *Water and Dreams* in 1983; and *La poétique de l'espace* (1958), which was translated and published as *The Poetics of Space* in 1964.

50   Also known as the Kwakwaka'wakw. One of their most important celebrations is a ceremonious feast called a potlatch, which is designed so the host can show off their wealth, sometimes by destroying things.

51   E. Graham Howe (1897–1975) was a British psychologist who helped found the Tavistock Clinic in London in 1920. Like Laing, Howe was interested in psychology in a non-medical way, employing practices and ideas from spirituality and existential philosophy. He was very important to Laing, whose quote, "Here is a master psychologist", is printed on the cover of the book Feldmár is quoting from *The Druid of Harley Street:*

The Spiritual Psychology of E. Graham Howe. Edited by William Stranger, the book was brought back into print and published in 2012 by North Atlantic Books, California. Original publication data is unknown.

[52] Marion Milner (1900–1998) was a British author and psychoanalyst who came up with a way of writing that has been called "introspective journaling". It is an early form, perhaps, of writing therapy and involves noting down day-to-day experiences and emotions, the thoughts that occur during those times and a particularly wide-open awareness of external sense stimulation. Feldmár met her during his time in London and is referring to two of her books here: *On Not Being Able to Paint* (1950) and *The Hands of the Living God* (1969), International Universities Press, New York.

[53] R.D. Laing's 12 recommended books are listed at the end of this book.

[54] The Holy Bible: King James Version. (1611). Ecclesiastes 11–12.

[55] See note 14, above, regarding Bowlby.

[56] Ballet Rambert was an English dance company founded by Dame Marie Rambert in 1920, now called Rambert Dance Company. Please see https://www.rambert.org.uk/about-us/our-history/ for more information.

[57] The Samaveda is the Veda of melodies and chants. It is an ancient Vedic Sanskrit text and part of the scriptures of Hinduism.

[58] *The Wisdom of Zhuang Zi on Daoism.* (2008). Translated with annotations and commentaries by Chung Wu, Peter Lang Publishing, New York.

[59] Euripides (484–406 BCE) was a Classical Greek playwright and tragedian. He is one of the most famous from that time, and his work continues to influence the theatre and playwrights to this day. A few of his more popular plays include *Electra, The Trojan Women, and Orestes.*

[60] Plato. *Apology* (B. Jowett Trans.). Public domain.

[61] T.S. Eliot. (1934). "Choruses from 'The Rock'", reprinted in *T.S. Eliot, Collected Poems 1909–1962* (1963). Houghton Mifflin Harcourt, New York.

[62] Giorgio Agamben. (2007). "Genius", in *Profanations* (J. Fort, Trans). Zone Books, New York.

[63] Feldmár met Gábor Karátson (1935–2015), a famous Hungarian writer, translator and painter, for the first time in 1959, when he, Feldmár, returned to Hungary for the first time since leaving in 1956. While there, he went to a meeting of the Anthroposophists, founded by Rudolf Steiner. One of the reasons Feldmár was there was because he wanted to meet Sándor Török. Török had written a children's book that Feldmár had loved as a child, and was an old classmate of Feldmár's father. It was Török who introduced Feldmár and Karátson initially, and they ended up becoming good friends.

[64] Szilvia Granasztói (b 1943) is Gábor Karátson's wife. Dávid and János are his sons.

[65] Wolf Wolfensberger. (1972). *The Principle of Normalization in Human Services*. National Institute on Mental Retardation, Canada.

[66] Ivan Illich. (1975). *Medical Nemesis: The Expropriation of Health*. Calder and Boyers, London.

[67] Attila József (1922). "Silent Evening Psalm". Babelmatrix.org (K. N. Ullrich, Trans.).

[68] Mullah Nasreddin. *The Jokes of Nasreddin Hodja* (Z. Hossain, Ed.). ABSURD's "Pure Wisdom" Series, Vol. 3, 2016. Mullah Nasreddin Hodja was a 13th-century satirist born in present-day Turkey.

[69] The essays by Freud that Feldmár was reading are "On Narcissism: An Introduction", which was originally published in German in 1914, and Mourning and Melancholia", which was originally published in 1917. *On Narcissism*, was published as a book in 2013 by Read Books. Both essays are available in English in *Sigmund Freud: Collected Papers*.

[70] Mihály Babits. (1904). "The Epilogue of the Lyric Poet". Babelmatrix.org (I. Tótfalusi, Trans.).

[71] Olga Nagy's book has not been translated into English. The original

Hungarian title is *Hősök, csalókák, ördögök*, and it was published in 1974.

[72] *A barna tehén fia*, by Feldmár and Büky, was published in Hungary, and only in Hungarian, by Jaffa Kft. in 2010.

[73] Mircea Eliade. (1964). *Shamanism: Archaic Techniques of Ecstasy* (W.R. Trask, Trans.). Princeton UP, New Jersey.

[74] Unknown poem by Kathleen Raine.

[75] Leonard Cohen. (1967). "The Stranger Song", *Songs of Leonard Cohen*. Columbia Records, New York.

A CONVERSATION WITH R.D. LAING

[1] R.D. Laing. (1976). *The Facts of Life: An Essay in Feelings, Facts and Fantasy.* Penguin, London.

[2] Ashley Montagu (1905–1999) was a British-American anthropologist, who studied and wrote on being human, on the fallacy of race, and on gender, to name a few topics. Feldmár is referring here to one of Montagu's books, *The Meaning of Love*, which was originally published in 1953 by Julian Press in New York.

[3] St Thomas Aquinas (1225–1274) was a very influential and important Italian theologian, friar and priest. He is known as one of the greatest Scholastic philosophers and was named a Doctor of the Church. He writes about knowledge and love in his *Summa Theologica*, originally published in 1485 in Latin. The English translation was published in 1917 by RCL Benziger, in Cincinnati, OH.

[4] Research indicates that "there is no knowledge without love" is actually a quote from St Bonaventure. However, there is evidence that St Thomas Aquinas said "love follows knowledge".

[5] George Chapman. (1968). *All Fools*. University of Nebraska Press, Lincoln.

[6] Paul Goodman (1911-1972) was an American author, sociologist, gay-rights activist, public intellectual and one of the founders of gestalt

therapy. One of his more famous books, which Feldmár is referring to here, is *Growing Up Absurd*, which came out in 1960 from Random House in New York.

[7] German: depict, shape, show, portray, represent, delineate, demonstrate.

[8] Bion developed his grid in order to create more precision in identifying, classifying, and generally discussing psychoanalytic material that is produced and experienced during the traditional hour-long session of psychoanalysis. He was attempting to create a sort of scientific theory of psychoanalysis by applying mathematic principles to the relations between thoughts/thinking and learning/growth. He did this by creating an x-axis of uses and functions attributed to thoughts and ideas and a y-axis of the evolution of thoughts and ideas. Later on in his work, he abandoned it and recognised its failure. For more information on the grid, please see his book *Elements of Psycho-analysis*, originally published in 1963 by Basic Books in New York.

[9] The Palo Alto School of Brief Therapy was founded in 1967 by Richard Fisch (1926–2011), John H. Weakland (1919–1995) and Paul Watzlawick (1921–2007). Their idea was to "cultivate a quick and effective therapy method, which we now know today as Problem-Solving Brief Therapy" (brieftherapycenter.org). The three of them also wrote a book together, *Change: Principles of Problem Formation and Problem Resolution*, which was published in 1974 by Norton, in New York. Gurdjieff's "way of blame" is taken from the Sufi history and practice of the Malamatiyya, an ancient mystical group that practised what became known as the way of blame. The name is from the Arabic word *malāmah*, which means "blame". They practised self-humility and were negatively critical of themselves and others. Feldmár has described it as a non-maternal form of tough love. For more information about Gurdjieff and Sufism, please see the book *Sufism and the Way of Blame: Hidden Sources of a Sacred Psychology*, by Yannis Toussulis, published in 2010 by Quest Books in Wheaton, IL, USA.

[10] R.D. Laing. (1979). *Sonnets*. Michael Joseph Ltd., London.

[11] Johan August Strindberg (1849–1912) was a well-known Swedish playwright, novelist, poet, essayist and painter. Göran Söderström, in his 1972 book *Strindberg och Bildkonsten* (which translates to *Strindberg and Visual Arts*, but has only been published in Swedish, by Forum), quotes Strindberg as saying: "Jealousy, holy feeling of purity of soul which despises being conjoined with another of the same sex by the mediation of another person. Jealousy, legitimate egoism, stemming from the preservation instinct of both self and race. The jealous one says to his rival: leave, deficient one; you will warm yourself in the flames I have ignited; you will breathe my breath from her mouth; you will imbibe my blood and you will remain my slave since it is my spirit that will control you through this woman, now become your master." This English translation comes from a note in an essay by Arnold Weinstein, called "Edvard Munch as Psychotherapist: 'The Horse Cure'", which was published in *Psychotherapy, Literature and the Visual and Performing Arts*, edited by Bruce Kirkcaldy and published in 2018 by Palgrave Macmillan in London.

[12] Kurt Gödel's (1906–1978) first incompleteness theorem, published in 1931, establishes that it is "impossible to use the axiomatic method to construct a formal system for any branch of mathematics containing arithmetic that will entail all of its truths" (https://www.britannica. com/topic/incompleteness-theorem#ref1107613). What this means is that the system itself will always be unable to actually prove every single true statement made about it, leading to a particular set of uncertainties.

[13] Lloyd deMause (1931–2020) was an American social thinker known for his work in the field of psychohistory. For more information about deMause's theory, please see *The History of Childhood*. (1974). Harper and Row, New York.

[14] Alan Watts (1915–1973) was a British philosopher, writer and speaker who was well known for bringing and popularising religions and spiritual

traditions from the East, like Buddhism (Zen and Tibetan), Hinduism, and Taoism by interpreting and basically translating them for Western audiences. For more information, please the website for the Alan Watts Organization at https://alanwatts.org.

[15] The Christian theory of equivocation, or really any equivocation, is a logical fallacy whereby an argument or statement is made with a term that changes meaning during the verbal exchange, conflating two meanings of the same word or phrase (homonyms). It is a strategy that enables the speaker to hide deception and thereby protect against accusation and punishment.

[16] The maxim "know thyself" is one of three phrases carved into a pillar at the entrance to the temple of Apollo at Delphi, in Greece. The other two, considered Delphic maxims, are "nothing to excess", and "certainty brings ruin."

[17] Laing, here, is asking about the relationship, as an equal one, an equation, meaning each side or party is equal (*adequatio*), between understanding/knowledge (*intellectu*) and things (*rei et*). He is playing with a quote from St. Thomas Aquinas, *"Veritas est adequatio rei et intellectus"*, meaning "Truth is an equation of, or equal to, knowledge and things."

[18] Gestalt therapy is a form of psychological therapy, developed by Fritz Perls (1893–1970), Paul Goodman (1911–1972), and Ralph Hefferline (1910–1974), that regards the patient's problem as a disruption in their total life system, or shape, including their network of relationships and other larger contexts, rather than an illness that is inside the patient. Transactional analysis is a method of therapy developed in the late 1950s by Eric Berne that analyses human relationships as a kind of series of transactions between self and other. This is done in order to determine the ego state of the patient as a basis for understanding their behaviour. The patient is then taught to alter their ego state as a way to solve emotional and relationship problems. For

more information, please see Berne's book *Games People Play: The Psychology of Human Relationships* (1964), published by Grove Press in New York.

[19] The Holy Bible: King James Version. (1611). Gospel of Matthew 7:7.

[20] Alexis Carrel. (1950). *The Voyage to Lourdes*. Harper & Brothers, New York.

[21] Primal therapy is a trauma-based therapy developed by Arthur Janov. See his book, *The Primal Scream. Primal Therapy: The Cure for Neurosis*. (1970). Dell Publishing, New York.

[22] Laing is referring to Halifax's 1979 book *Shamanic Voices*, published by EP Dutton, in Boston.

[23] Humphry Osmond (1917–2004) was a British psychoanalyst who coined the term "psychedelic" in 1958. He conducted experiments with LSD and other psychedelic drugs, working with Abram Hoffer, Aldous Huxley, Timothy Leary and others. He is also well known for his experiments and work attempting to cure alcoholics with LSD therapy. Later, after continuing his psychedelic research grew more difficult, he became the director of the Bureau of Research in Neurology and Psychiatry at the New Jersey Neuro-Psychiatric Institute in Princeton. There, he worked with Bernard S. Aaronson, doing hypnosis research and experiments. They co-authored a book together, called *Psychedelics: The Uses and Implications of Hallucinogenic Drugs* (1970), published by Anchor Books, in New York. While the documentary film Laing refers to is presently unknown, one of the essays published in *Psychedelics* by Aaronson, "Some Hypnotic Analogues to the Psychedelic State", describes hypnotic experiments using a metronome, much like what Laing describes here.

SHAMANISM, HEALING AND R.D. LAING

* From Salman Raschid (Ed.) (2005) *R.D. Laing: Contemporary Perspectives*. Free Association Books, London.

1. "The House of Rimmon" or "to bow in the House of Rimmon" means to yield one's beliefs or principles in order to conform to the rules of the house. The phrase is from the Hebrew Bible, 2 Kings 5 18, and refers to the Syrian god Rimmon (known elsewhere as Baal or Ramanu).

2. Margaret J Field. (1962). *Search for Security: An Ethno-psychiatric Study of Rural Ghana*. Northwestern University Press, Illinois.

3. See note 73 in the "Journal Entries" section above, regarding Mircea Eliade's book on shamanism.

4. Samuel Taylor Coleridge (1772–1834) was an English poet, philosopher, and theologian who is credited, along with his friend William Wordsworth, for founding the Romantic movement that swept across the UK and much of Europe. While the exact source of Huxley's paraphrase is not known, it is likely from one of the following works by Coleridge: *Lay Sermons* (1817), *Aids to Reflection* (1825) or *The Constitution of Church and State* (1830).

5. Coventry Patmore (1823–1896) was a British Victorian poet and critic. Huxley's quote is from Patmore's book, *The Rod, the Root and the Flower*, published in 1950 by Grey Walls, in London.

6. Lucien Lévy-Bruhl (1857–1939) was a French philosopher and scholar whose main field of work ended up being what is referred to as the "mentality of primitive peoples". He is credited with furthering the pursuit of anthropology by promoting the budding fields of sociology and ethnography. Werner Heisenberg (1901–1976) was a German theoretical physicist who is known for coming up with the uncertainty principle and founding the field of quantum mechanics, for which he won the Nobel Prize in 1932.

7. Jacob Boehme (1575–1624) was a German philosopher, Christian mystic and Lutheran Protestant theologian. His best-known work, also called his

351

masterwork, is *Signatura Rerum*, or *The Signature of All Things*, originally published in High Dutch in 1622 and translated by John Ellistone in 1651. Huxley is quoting from Chapter 9 of this book.

[8] Knud Rasmussen (1879–1933) was a Greenlandic/Dutch explorer, anthropologist and ethnologist. He spent most of his time living with and studying multiple tribes across the northern arctic expanse, from Greenland to the Bering Strait. The exact source of Huxley's quote is not known, but it may be in one of these two books by Rasmussen: *The People of the Polar North*. (1908). Kegan Paul, Trench, Trübner & Co. Ltd., London, or *Greenland by the Polar Sea: The Story of the Thule Expedition from Melville Bay to Cape Morris Jesup*. (1921). W. Heinemann, London.

[9] Hubert Butler. (1972). *Ten Thousand Saints: A Study of Irish and European Origins*. Wellbrook Press, Kilkenny, Ireland.

[10] Francis Huxley. (1969). *The Invisibles: Voodoo Gods in Haiti*. McGraw Hill, New York.

[11] Carl Rogers (1902–1987) was a famous American psychologist who furthered and promoted client-centred therapy. He is widely acknowledged as one of the founders of humanistic psychology. The encounter between Laing and Rogers is described by Charles Elliot in "Carl Rogers encounters R.D. Laing." (1978). *Self & Society: An International Journal for Humanistic Psychology, (6)*10, 360–362.

[12] Martin Buber. (1965). *The Knowledge of Man: Selected Essays by Martin Buber*. Harper & Row, New York.

[13] Peter Mezan, is a psychoanalyst working in New York and an assistant clinical professor of psychiatry at Mount Sinai Hospital. Earlier in his career, he lived in London and worked with Laing and the Philadelphia Association. He lectured on family systems for the PA and helped introduce Laing and his ideas to the American public.

FANTASY AND REALITY

[1] From the *Stanford Encyclopedia of Philosophy*: "The Aristotelian sciences divide into three: (i) theoretical, (ii) practical, and (iii) productive. The principles of division are straightforward: theoretical science seeks knowledge for its own sake; practical science concerns conduct and goodness in action, both individual and societal; and productive science aims at the creation of beautiful or useful objects." https://plato.stanford.edu/ entries/aristotle/.

[2] Both Giordano Bruno (1548–1600) and Galileo Galilei (1564–1642) were tried and convicted of heresy, though with Galilei it was only his heliocentric model of the universe that got him into trouble, whereas with Bruno, that was only part of it. Bruno ended up with 130 charges against him. Galilei was found guilty only of mid-level heresy.

[3] *Novum Organon*, or *New Instrument*, was written by Francis Bacon in Latin, and published in England in 1620. See *The New Organon*. (2000). (M. Silverthorne, Trans.). (L. Jardine, Ed.). Cambridge UP, UK.

[4] The Holy Bible: King James Version. (1611). Romans, 5:13.

[5] R.D. Laing. (1967). *The Politics of Experience and the Bird of Paradise*. Penguin Books, UK. The quote is from Chapter 2, "The Psychotherapeutic Experience", which was published earlier, in 1965, as "Practice and Theory: The Present Situation", in the journal *Psychotherapy and Psychosomatics*.

[6] Léopold (Lipót) Szondi (1893–1986) was a Hungarian psychiatrist, psychoanalyst, and professor of psychology. He is known for coming up with fate analysis and creating the Szondi test. For more information about Szondi and his work, please see the website for The Szondi Institute, at https://szondi.ch/?lang=en.

[7] Sándor Ferenczi (1873–1933) was a Hungarian psychoanalyst and was, initially, a close colleague and friend of Sigmund Freud. It was only later in his life that distance grew between them and their relationship deteriorated. Ferenczi founded the Hungarian Psychoanalytic Society and

was the cornerstone of the Budapest School of Psychoanalysis. Feldmár's paraphrase is from Ferenczi's book, *The Clinical Diary of Sándor Ferenczi* (M. Balint and N. Z. Jackson, Trans.) (J. Dupont, Ed.), published in 1988 by Harvard University Press.

[8] Jerzy Kosinski (1933–1991) was a Jewish Polish-American writer and novelist. He survived World War II and emigrated to the US. Some of his novels became quite famous and were made into movies, though there was some controversy over plagiarism. He died by suicide in New York. The source for what Feldmár says is an interview Kosinski did for the Paris Review in 1972: "Jerzy Kosinski, The Art of Fiction No. 46." *The Paris Review*, (*Summer*)54. The interviewers are George Plimpton and Rocco Landesman.

[9] Sigmund Freud. (1949). *An Outline of Psychoanalysis*. Hogarth Press, London.

[10] This course took place during the fall of 1967 at the University of Western Ontario, right after Feldmár had begun working with Zenon Pylyshyn.

[11] William S. Burroughs. (1959). *Naked Lunch*. Grove Press, New York.

[12] Daniel Paul Schreber. (1988). *Memoirs of My Nervous Illness (1903)*. (I. MacAlpine and R.A. Hunter, Trans. and Eds.) Harvard UP, Cambridge, MA. Freud's analysis of Schreber was published as "The Case of Schreber" in 1958 in Volume 12 (1911–1913) of *The Standard Edition of the Complete Psychological Works of Freud*, by The Hogarth Press in London.

[13] E. E. Cummings. (2013). *E. E. Cummings: Complete Poems 1904–1962*. Liveright, New York.

[14] David Bakan. (1966). *The Duality of Human Existence: Isolation and Communion in Western Man*. Beacon Press, Boston.

[15] Emmanuel Levinas. (1969). *Totality and Infinity*. (A. Lingis, Trans.). Duquesne UP, Pittsburgh.

[16] Georg Wilhelm Friedrich Hegel (1770–1831) was a German philosopher and one of the last great system-builders. He developed a style or scheme for arguing called "dialectics", which is still important today. See Hegel's

books *Lectures on Aesthetics* (1975). (T.M. Knox, Trans.) Clarendon Press, Oxford; and *Phenomenology of Spirit.* (1977). (A.V. Miller, Trans.). Clarendon Press, Oxford. Michel Foucault (1926–1984) was a French philosopher, critic, activist and historian. See his books *The Order of Things: An Archaeology of the Human Sciences* (1970. Tavistock, London); *Discipline and Punish: The Birth of Prison* (1977. Pantheon Books, New York); and *The History of Sexuality,* a four-volume work published in English from 1978 to 2018, initially by Pantheon Books in New York. Slavoj Žižek (b 1949) is a Slovenian philosopher whose main interests include ideology, Marxism, political philosophy, psychoanalysis and cultural studies. See his books *The Sublime Object of Ideology* (1989. Verso Books, London); and *Plague of Fantasies* (1997. Verso Books, London).

[17] Josef Švejk is the protagonist of several humorous short stories and an unfinished satirical novel by Czech author Jaroslav Hašek, published from 1921–1923. Švejk has become a symbol of passive resistance, liberty and the Czech national character. For more information, please see Cecil Parrott's book *Jaroslav Hašek: A Study of Švejk and the Short Stories* (1982). Cambridge University Press, UK.

[18] David Smail (1938–2014) was a British psychologist who favoured the consideration of social materialism in analysing psychological distress. Later in his career and life, he began to doubt the entire enterprise of psychology. The three things a therapist can do to help someone, which Feldmár writes about here, is from Smail's 1993 book *The Origins of Unhappiness: A New Understanding of Personal Distress,* published by HarperCollins in New York.

[19] Jean-Paul Sartre (1905–1980) was a French philosopher, playwright, novelist, screenwriter, political activist, biographer and literary critic. He is known for being prominent in the existential and phenomenological branches of philosophy. For more information and reading on Sartre's understanding of praxis and process, please see R.D. Laing and D. G.

Cooper's 1964 book, *Reason and Violence,* originally published by Tavistock, in London, and Sartre's 1960 book, *Critique of Dialectical Reason,* first published in English in 1976 (A. Sheridan-Smith, Trans.) by New Left Books, London.

[20] These are recurring elements in Hungarian folk tales.

[21] In Hungary, on Christmas Eve, Santa Claus gives good children candy or chocolate and naughty children birch or coal.

[22] The anecdote that Feldmár writes about is from Jung's 1961 book, *Memories, Dreams, Reflections,* originally published in English in 1963 (R. and C. Wilson, Trans.) by Random House in New York.

[23] This is Feldmár's translation of Ákos Fodor's poem, *"Vigasz"* [Consolation], from *Buddha Weimarban* [Buddha in Weimar], published in 2002 in Hungary.

[24] See note 52 in the "Journal Entries" section above, regarding Marion Milner.

[25] Susan Sontag. (1978). *Illness as Metaphor.* Farrar, Straus & Giroux, New York.

[26] Jacques Lacan (1901–1981) was a prominent and controversial French psychoanalyst and psychiatrist. His work continues to be important and influential, both for the intellectual history of France and the fields of psychology and psychoanalysis. One of his more important theories is his concept of the Real, something he wrote about and developed throughout his work. For more information, please see his lecture "The Symbolic, the Imaginary, and the Real," which he presented on July 8, 1953, and which marked the beginning of his public teaching. It is in his book, *On the Names-of-the-Father,* translated by Bruce Fink and published in 2013 by Polity Press, in Cambridge, UK. The original French, *Des noms-du-père* was published in 2005 by Editions du Seuil in Paris.

[27] Ludwig Wittgenstein. (1922). *The Tractatus Logico-Philosophicus* (F. P. Ramsey and C. K. Ogden, Trans.). Harcourt, Brace & Company, New York.

[28] Epictetus writes, "Remember that the door is open. Don't be more cowardly than children, but just as they say, when the game is no longer fun for them, 'I won't play anymore,' you too, when things seem that way to you, say, 'I won't play anymore,' and leave, but if you remain, don't complain," in *Discourses* 1.24.20. And Seneca writes, in Letter 58, popularly called "On Being", "If I find out that the pain must always be endured, I shall depart, not because of the pain but because it will be a hindrance to me as regards all my reasons for living. He who dies just because he is in pain is a weakling, a coward; but he who lives merely to brave out this pain, is a fool," which can be found in *The Epistles of Lucius Annæus Seneca*, originally published in 65CE, and first published in English in 1786 (T. Morell, Trans.) by Oxford University.

[29] For Heidegger, *vorhanden* or "present-at-hand" and *zuhanden* or "ready-to-hand" are modes of being.

[30] Victor E. Frankl (1905–1997) was a Jewish Austrian neurologist, psychiatrist and philosopher who survived the Holocaust. He developed and promoted what he called logotherapy, which comes from his belief that the search for meaning, for the meaning of life, is the main human motivation. For more information, please see Frankl's 1946 book *Man's Search for Meaning: An Introduction to Logotherapy* which was published in English in 1959 (I. Lasch, Trans.) by Beacon Press in Boston.

[31] Mihaly Csikszentmihalyi (b 1934) is a Hungarian-American psychologist. He is best known and recognised for his identification of the mental state that is highly focused towards the composition or production of something. Csikszentmihalyi named this state "flow". For more information, please see his 1990 book, *Flow*, published by Harper & Row in New York.

[32] Duncan Blewett (1920–2007) was a Canadian psychologist, teacher and researcher. For more information about the LSD experiment Feldmár

references here, please see Blewett's 1969 book, *The Frontiers of Being: Dynamics of Love and Awareness*, published by Award Books, Canada.

33 *Plaisir* can be translated as obvious pleasure or enjoyment. *Jouissance* is more difficult to translate into English and refers to a kind of hidden, inner, and deep pleasure. In French, *plaisir* is used for male orgasm and *jouissance* for female orgasm.

34 Georges Devereux (1908–1985) was a Hungarian-French ethnologist, anthropologist and psychiatrist. He is often considered the founder of ethnopsychiatry. Throughout his career, he spent approximately thirty years living, studying and working in the US, where he got his ethnology degree and did fieldwork with multiple indigenous tribes. For more information on the story Feldmár recounts here, please see Devereux's 1967 book, *From Anxiety to Method in the Behavioral Sciences*, published by Mouton in The Hague.

35 Quote from Hungary's national poet, Sándor Petőfi, from the poem *Nemzeti Dal* [Song of the Nation].

36 Gregory Bateson. (1991). *A Sacred Unity: Further Steps to an Ecology of Mind* (R. Donaldson, Ed.). HarperCollins, New York.

37 Jean-Paul Sartre. (1992). *Notebooks for an Ethics* (D. Pellauer, Trans.). University of Chicago Press, Chicago. Originally published as *Cahiers pour une morale* in 1983, by Gallimard in Paris.

38 See note 15, above, regarding Levinas source.

39 D. W. Winnicott. (1986). *Babies and Their Mothers*. Addison-Wesley, Boston. The book was published posthumously with materials culled from the estate, as Winnicott died in 1971.

40 The Holy Bible: King James Version. (1611). Gospel of Matthew 26:42.

41 For more information about the anecdote Feldmár is referring to, please see Charles J. Stivale's essay, "Horny Dudes: Guy de Maupassant and the Masculine *Feuille de rose*", published in *L'Esprit Créateur*, *43*(3), 57-67.

About the Author

Andrew Feldmár is a Vancouver-based psychologist and psychotherapist. His approach to therapy seeks to reconnect patients to the joys of everyday life through relying on loving, living relationships, rather than the alienation of the classical doctor–patient relationship. He was born in Hungary during WWII (1940), and after the 1956 revolution was defeated, he immigrated to Canada on his own at the age of 16. He graduated with honors from the University of Toronto with a BA in mathematics, physics, and chemistry, as well as an MA in psychology from the University of Western Ontario. He has been a psychotherapist since 1969.

During 1974–1975, he spent a year in London, England, intensively studying and training in the practice of psychotherapy under the renowned and controversial Scottish psychiatrist, R.D. Laing. During this year, he also studied with Francis Huxley (the anthropology of healing), John Heaton (existential psychotherapy), Hugh Crawford (community therapy), and Leon Redler (spiritual emergency). These relationships became lifelong friendships. Feldmár also worked with one of the founders of transpersonal psychology, Stanislav Grof at the Esalen Institute in California. He gained further experience in the field while volunteering at Hollywood Hospital in New Westminster, where LSD was legally used for research and therapy. He gained experience in brief psychotherapy in Palo Alto in the research group of Paul Watzlawick.

He has taught, lectured, and led workshops at Simon Fraser University (SFU), The University of British Columbia (UBC), Emily Carr University, and Douglas College. In 1989, he was a guest on a 3-part CBC Ideas radio series entitled *R.D. Laing Today*. He has also worked as a consultant in both television and film (e.g., Showcase's Kink series, *Neurons to Nirvana: The Great Medicines*). Other career highlights include work with the United Nations; founding the Integra Households Association, a non-profit charity working with those in extreme mental distress; and Third Mind Productions, a film production company that went on to turn out the 1987 film, *Did You Used to Be R.D. Laing?*

He has also worked extensively overseas, mainly in Hungary, where he has published over 30 books. His first book, *The Rainbow of States of Consciousness*, is now in its third edition. Two organisations have been set up in Hungary, inspired by Feldmár. The Soteria Foundation was established in 1995 and became a pioneer of community psychiatric care in the country. In 2006, his colleagues and friends founded the Feldmár Institute, in Budapest, in order to popularise his theoretical and practical approach to psychotherapy.

He is well-known to international audiences in the field of psychedelic-assisted psychotherapy, having presented at numerous conferences on the subject. He took part in a research study sponsored by MAPS Canada in 2008 to demonstrate the efficacy of MDMA as an adjunct to psychotherapy in patients with severe PTSD. He was also a mentor in California's Psychedelic-Assisted Therapies and Research program.